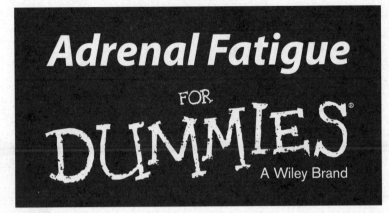

by Dr. Richard Snyder, DO,
and Wendy Jo Peterson, MS, RD

Foreword by Martie Whittekin, CCN

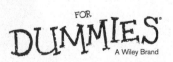

Adrenal Fatigue For Dummies®

Published by: **John Wiley & Sons, Inc.,** 111 River Street, Hoboken, NJ 07030-5774, www.wiley.com

For general information on our other products and services, please contact our Customer Care Department within the U.S. at 877-762-2974, outside the U.S. at 317-572-3993, or fax 317-572-4002. For technical support, please visit www.wiley.com/techsupport.

Wiley publishes in a variety of print and electronic formats and by print-on-demand. Some material included with standard print versions of this book may not be included in e-books or in print-on-demand. If this book refers to media such as a CD or DVD that is not included in the version you purchased, you may download this material at http://booksupport.wiley.com. For more information about Wiley products, visit www.wiley.com.

Library of Congress Control Number: 2013954225

ISBN 978-1-118-61580-5 (pbk); ISBN 978-1-118-61569-0 (ebk); ISBN 978-1-118-61578-2 (ebk)

Manufactured in the United States of America

10 9 8 7 6 5 4 3 2

Contents at a Glance

Recipes at a Glance

Desserts and Snacks

Table of Contents

Foreword

I was eager to interview Dr. Rich Snyder about adrenal fatigue on my radio show because I've long thought it an important issue. He did for my listeners what he and coauthor Wendy Jo Peterson have done in this book: translate complex issues into lay terms. They distilled their impressive research into a guide so practical that it contains recipes. Every reader can learn to feel better, and lives will surely be saved because readers can relieve their symptoms by coming to the aid of their adrenal glands instead of resorting to worrisome medications.

In writing a book about acid reflux, I was shocked that clever marketing has — by convincing Americans that heartburn requires acid-blocking drugs — boosted annual sales of the medications to more than $14 billion. Acid-blockers relieve pain by stopping normal digestion at the risk of potentially life-threatening side effects. And ironically, the acid-suppression approach ignores the fact that *insufficient* stomach acid is quite often the cause of the reflux.

It now seems acceptable to assume that any health complaint is due to the deficiency of a prescription drug. For example, if a person is depressed, we're told that he or she needs an antidepressant drug (or two). Seldom do we hear that the cause might be adrenal fatigue, which the antidepressant won't fix. The automatic response to high blood pressure is hypertension medication. But again, if an adrenal problem is the cause, addressing it would be a safer, more fundamental solution. Likewise, we see popular drugs for insomnia, anxiety, sexual dysfunction, osteoporosis, and back pain — all conditions that might also be due to stressed adrenals. Although medication may be necessary to manage symptoms (at least temporarily), it carries the risk of side effects and isn't a good substitute for finding the root cause of the problem and fixing it.

Similarly, consumers appear to think that they're tired because they're a quart low on coffee. Little do they suspect that their fatigue (as well as the extra inches around their middles) may be related to stressed-out adrenal glands. Of greater concern is the fact that, like other unaddressed imbalances, unresolved adrenal distress can lead to diabetes and other serious health problems over time.

But then, who can blame anyone for ignoring a body part that they can't see and that doesn't call attention to itself? There are no instantly associated clues like direct pain or a dash to the bathroom. *Adrenal Fatigue For Dummies* provides clues that one's adrenal glands may be overworked as well as specific steps for confirming a problem and treating it.

We shouldn't be deterred by mainstream medicine's rather dismissive attitude about the concept of adrenal fatigue. There's certainly a wealth of supporting science and a huge number of successes in the clinical experience of integrative medical practices. However, except in naturopathic medical schools, little attention may be given to the subject during doctor training. Perhaps an even bigger issue is that third-party payers like insurance companies and government programs don't typically reimburse for the time required to do the detective work of tracking down and resolving these subtle imbalances.

Fortunately, armed with the facts in *Adrenal Fatigue For Dummies,* if readers haven't solved their problems independently, they can be respectful advocates for themselves when they visit their doctor. The right physician will listen and may even want to read the book, which also contains a great deal of helpful general information about how diet and lifestyle affect health. Happily, most all of Dr. Snyder's nature-based recommendations and Wendy Jo's recipes and nutrition tips will help not only the adrenals but also many other body systems at the same time. Natural approaches are like that — they offer fringe benefits instead of side effects.

Martie Whittekin, CCN
Syndicated radio host
Author of *Natural Alternatives to Nexium, Maalox, Tagamet, Prilosec & Other Acid Blockers*

Introduction

Adrenal fatigue is one of the most commonly misunderstood conditions in modern healthcare. It often goes undiagnosed, and therefore millions of people suffer from it. So if *you* have adrenal fatigue, you're not alone.

Adrenal fatigue isn't in the history books. It's known as a "disease of modern life."

You've likely felt tired and fatigued for a long time. Maybe you've visited healthcare providers who haven't heard of adrenal fatigue and others who don't believe it exists. Tell that to your body! You know that what you're going through isn't all in your head. Yes, this condition exists, and no, you aren't crazy.

Don't fret — we wrote this book for people suffering from adrenal fatigue. Having adrenal fatigue that has either been undiagnosed or misdiagnosed has no doubt been a frustrating and draining experience for you, but that's about to come to an end. We wrote this book to take the mystery out of adrenal fatigue. We wanted to put a name to some of the symptoms that you're suffering from.

In addition to describing adrenal fatigue, we provide you with the information you need to help you manage the condition. We also want to provide you with support and encouragement.

This book is about a journey to help you take your life back. We want you to eliminate any negativity and embrace positivity. Treating adrenal fatigue is the only way you'll be able to move forward in your life, and you'll be glad for that!

About This Book

Adrenal Fatigue For Dummies puts a lot of good information in 20 chapters. Each chapter stands on its own, so you can reference any chapters you need to in any order. The book has the following features:

- ✔ **Easy-to-understand language:** It's written in plain English. There's little medical jargon, and this book is by no means a medical reference book.

  In some instances, we use italics to highlight medical terms, diseases, and bacteria and fungus names you should know. Drug names appear with the generic name first, followed by a brand name.

✔ **Coverage of all aspects of adrenal fatigue:** We include symptoms, diagnosis, and treatment.

✔ **References to research:** A lot of current research investigates conditions related to adrenal health. And in the world of nutrition, researchers make new discoveries about the beneficial natural chemicals in food every day. One of our goals is to give you as much up-to-date information as possible.

✔ **Info on what *not* to do in addition to what to do:** Knowing what to do (and when to do it) is very important, of course, but sometimes it's just as important to know when to avoid a food, a medicine, or an activity.

✔ **Insight of both a physician and a nutritionist:** You're getting firsthand clinical information from a doctor who sees patients as well as from a nutritionist. Nutrition is so important that we dedicate several chapters to this aspect of healing.

✔ **Recipes:** Coauthor Wendy Jo offers pages of recipes to help you give your adrenal glands the nutritional boost they need.

✔ **Text that isn't boring (we hope):** Because this is a *For Dummies* book, you can count on it being lively, light, and easy to read.

Feel free to skip anything marked with the Technical Stuff icon as well as the sidebars (those chunks of text that appear in shaded boxes). They aren't necessary for understanding, diagnosing, or treating adrenal fatigue.

Some web addresses may break across two lines of text. If you're reading this book in print and want to visit one of these web pages, pretend the line break doesn't exist and key in the web address exactly as it's noted in the text. If you're reading this as an e-book, you've got it easy — just select the web address to go directly to the web page.

Foolish Assumptions

In writing this book, we had to make a few assumptions about you:

✔ You think you have some symptoms of adrenal fatigue but haven't been diagnosed, and you want more information. Or you've been diagnosed with adrenal fatigue, but you want more details about how to manage and treat it.

✔ You want an integrative/holistic approach to treating adrenal fatigue, so you're interested in finding out more about natural therapies.

✔ You're starving to discover how to boost your adrenal health through nutrition, which comes from eating the right foods and taking the right dietary supplements.

Icons Used in This Book

The little images in the margins of this book draw your attention to different nuggets of information. We use the following icons:

 A Remember icon calls out important adrenal fatigue information that needs to stay with you.

 A Tip is a suggestion or a recommendation. It's a quick hint concerning adrenal fatigue.

A Warning describes a serious situation in which you should exercise care and perhaps seek additional advice. Numerous diagnostic scenarios can be critical to your well-being, and you need to be aware of them.

At times, we have to unload a little medical jargon on you or share some other interesting yet nonessential information. Reading these items isn't mandatory. That being said, they provide some insight and doctor talk about adrenal fatigue.

Beyond the Book

In addition to the material in the book you're reading right now, we've put some access-anywhere extras out on the web. For some key facts about adrenal fatigue symptoms and management, check out the free Cheat Sheet at www.dummies.com/cheatsheet/adrenalfatigue. Also, be sure to visit www.dummies.com/extras/adrenalfatigue for free articles about connecting intestinal health to adrenal fatigue, reducing work stress to ease adrenal fatigue, and more.

Where to Go From Here

In theory, you can read any chapters in this book in any order. However, it's a good idea to start with Part I, which covers the basics of adrenal fatigue (such as adrenal gland anatomy, adrenal fatigue symptoms, and so on). Then use the table of contents and index to jump to whichever topics interest you most.

Not only will you gain insight into adrenal fatigue, but you'll also be able to formulate a personalized nutrition and treatment plan with the guidance of your healthcare provider. That plan will get you where you want to go. You need to be your own advocate for this condition, and we hope that this book will be a springboard for you in that direction.

Part I
Getting Started with Adrenal Fatigue

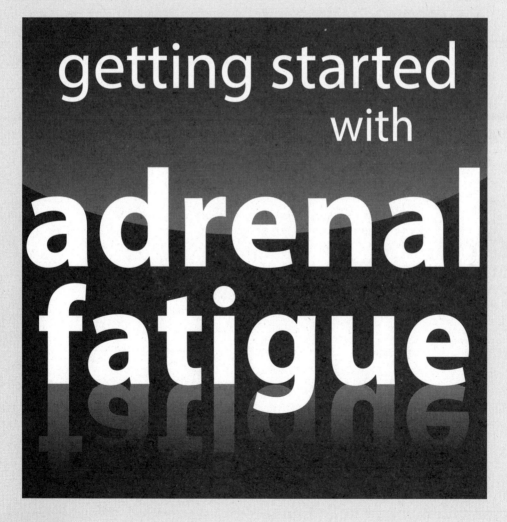

getting started
with
adrenal
fatigue

Visit www.dummies.com for great (and free!) Dummies content online.

In this part...

- Discover what adrenal fatigue is (and what it isn't). Healthcare providers underdiagnose adrenal fatigue, so it's important to know the factors that may lead to adrenal fatigue, the stages of adrenal fatigue, and similar syndromes.

- Understand what the adrenal glands do and how they work. Find out about their anatomy, hormone production, regulation of blood pressure and blood chemistry, pH balance, and interaction with other body parts.

- Recognize the symptoms of adrenal fatigue. They relate to vital signs, blood sugar levels, salt cravings, feeling sick and tired, bowel and bladder irritation, brain fog, depression, and more.

- Complete a questionnaire to figure out your chances of having adrenal fatigue, and understand the testing that's done to diagnose the condition. These tests cover hormones, acid-base balance, inflammation, and infection.

Chapter 1

Facing Adrenal Fatigue

*I*f you're reading this book, you're likely sick and tired of feeling sick and tired, and you want to know why you feel that way. You know something isn't right, and you're looking for reasons as to why you feel so run down. You may have grown frustrated with your healthcare providers' inability to pinpoint why you don't feel right. You suspect that you have adrenal fatigue.

You can take solace in the fact that thousands of people are experiencing similar symptoms and have complaints similar to yours. This book helps you understand what adrenal fatigue is, examines its causes, and explores how to evaluate and treat this condition.

Focusing on Adrenal Gland Function

The adrenal glands are two organs of the body that people don't often think about. Yet they're vital to your health and well-being because they do so much. To fully understand how adrenal fatigue can affect your health, you first need to understand the many functions of the adrenal glands.

You can think of the adrenal glands as regulators of the human body, overseeing many processes. Your adrenal glands are important in regulating blood pressure and acid-base balance. They're also important in the production of many hormones, which are crucial in the evaluation and management of adrenal fatigue. Examples of the hormones that your adrenal glands secrete include aldosterone, the sex hormones (namely, androstenedione, dehydroepiandros-terone [DHEA], and pregnenolone), and the all-important cortisol. We cover the fundamentals of adrenal gland structure and function in Chapter 2.

Figuring Out Adrenal Fatigue Factors, Stages, and Symptoms

If you were to keep your car running 24/7 and never shut it off, your engine would simply burn out. If you never had your car tuned up, never changed your oil, and used lower octane gas, then your engine would be at a much higher risk of burning out faster. Similarly, *adrenal fatigue* occurs when the adrenal glands are constantly working and never have time to rest and recover. Stimulated by acidity, inflammation, and chronic illness, the adrenal glands secrete way more cortisol than they should.

Cortisol is a necessary hormone. In the setting of an acute injury or illness, this hormone is important in turning off the acute inflammatory process when it's no longer needed. However, in chronic illness and chronic inflammation, the adrenal glands continue to produce cortisol. Over time, the adrenal glands become so fatigued that they aren't able to produce enough of the hormones that the body needs to function on a daily basis, such as cortisol and aldosterone.

A number of factors may lead to adrenal fatigue: heredity, stressors early in life, medication effects, and environmental and psychological factors. In Chapter 3, you read more about these factors, the stages of adrenal fatigue, and the differences between adrenal fatigue and other adrenal-related syndromes, including Cushing's syndrome and Addison's disease.

The best patients are those who are attuned to their bodies. Often, a patient with adrenal fatigue can have one or many symptoms, including constant fatigue that doesn't get better, even with a good night's sleep. You may notice increasing dizziness or lightheadedness if you stand up too quickly. You may notice that your blood pressure is lower than usual. You may find yourself craving salt more. In Chapter 4, you read about many of the typical and atypical symptoms that someone with adrenal fatigue can experience.

Being Tested for Adrenal Fatigue

Proper testing for adrenal fatigue is important to see whether you need supplementation with the hormones you read about in Chapter 2, including cortisol, aldosterone, and sex hormones like DHEA.

But the testing of adrenal gland function involves much more than simply measuring the levels of hormones in your blood. Salivary testing is much more accurate than blood testing. In addition, your healthcare provider should look for causes of adrenal fatigue by measuring toxin levels, searching for food sensitivities, and looking for potential causes of inflammation. See Chapter 5 for more information on being tested for adrenal fatigue.

Digging Deeper into Potential Triggers

After you recognize the symptoms of adrenal fatigue, you want to determine its causes. Major causes include chronic stress, lack of sleep, chronic inflammation, acidity, poor nutrition, and impaired intestinal health. You can't begin to treat adrenal fatigue without treating these underlying conditions. This section gives you a brief overview of these specific trigger factors; in Part II, you read about them in depth.

Adrenal fatigue is often a result of multiple causes that occur simultaneously. For example, someone with a chronic illness likely suffers from increased inflammation, has poor nutrition, lacks quality sleep, and has an unhealthy intestinal tract.

Stressing out and sleeping poorly

In Chapter 6, you read about the many kinds of stress people in modern times have to deal with (the adrenal glands have to deal with these multiple stresses as well). These include emotional stressors, physical stressors, and other stressors that you may not even be aware of, including electromagnetic stress.

Chapter 6 also discusses how people sleep poorly and how they can sleep better. Notice we didn't say sleep *longer*. Certainly, getting seven to eight hours of good quality sleep each night is important, but even if you get the requisite number of hours, you still may be sleeping badly. Sleeping *better* involves improving both sleep quantity and sleep quality.

Being inflamed and out of balance

Inflammation often goes hand in hand with adrenal fatigue, so it's important to be aware of inflammation's potential triggers. Chapter 7 covers some of those triggers, including chronic illnesses such as rheumatoid arthritis, lupus, fibromyalgia syndrome, Lyme disease, thyroid dysfunction, and celiac disease.

Another potent trigger of adrenal fatigue is acidosis. The kidneys and adrenal glands can get extremely stressed out trying to deal with the daily acid load that people impose on them each day through the Western diet and conditions such as diabetes. See Chapter 7 for information on acidosis.

Handling nutrition issues

Proper nutrition is vital to combating adrenal fatigue. The food choices you make can directly affect the health of your intestines, and the intestines are the root of all chronic illness and inflammation. If you have a healthy gut, then the amount of inflammation in your body is likely minimal. A diet high in sugar and processed foods, on the other hand, can increase the risk of yeast overgrowth in the intestine, inciting even more inflammation. Eating foods that you may be sensitive to or even allergic to can also have toxic and inflammatory effects on your body.

You should also be aware of the role nutrient deficiencies play in the perpetuation of total body inflammation and adrenal stress. You may eat three meals a day but still be severely malnourished. Deficiencies in minerals and vitamins can cause issues with your health.

Chapter 8 has the lowdown on the role that nutrition plays in adrenal fatigue.

Getting Treated

Everyone is different, and not everyone manifests symptoms of adrenal fatigue the same way. So although the treatment of adrenal fatigue is complex and multifaceted, it is (and should be) personalized to fit your particular health concerns and health needs. In Part III, we get to the nitty-gritty of treating adrenal fatigue.

Finding a practitioner

One of the most challenging aspects of diagnosing and treating adrenal fatigue is finding a good healthcare provider who has an understanding of this condition. Your current doctor or healthcare provider may not even be aware of the condition or give credence to its existence. In Chapter 9, you read about healthcare practitioners who have expertise not only in recognizing the condition but also in diagnosing and treating it. Examples include naturopathic physicians, holistic medical physicians, and other healthcare practitioners certified in anti-aging medicine.

Nutritionists are also invaluable because the first line of defense in improving your adrenal health is nutrition. Changing how you eat and choosing the right foods can make your adrenal glands stronger and allow you to feel better. It's no accident that a nutritionist, Wendy Jo Peterson, is a coauthor of this book. She's restored thousands of people to better health and a fuller life.

Chapter 9 explores a team approach to your health and wellness care. Maintaining communication and holding yourself accountable for changes you need to make are key to your success.

Making the most of medications and hormone supplements

After you identify one or more healthcare providers to work with, you can begin to talk about the treatment of adrenal fatigue. Chapter 10 reviews some of the medications that your practitioner may prescribe to help raise your blood pressure and keep it in an acceptable range.

Chapter 10 also explores some of the hormones that your healthcare provider may prescribe to treat adrenal fatigue, including hydrocortisone and fludrocortisone. The results of testing (see Chapter 5) determine whether you need to be on supplements along with these hormones. We also discuss hormone replacement with bioidentical hormones such as estrogen, progesterone, and DHEA.

Because the treatment of adrenal fatigue is personalized, your treatment plan may not require bioidentical hormone replacement. The plan for treatment depends on the levels of your hormones.

Considering alternative treatments

In your journey to overcome adrenal fatigue, supplementing your diet with extra nutrients can make all the difference, but you need to be careful. Treatment should not only support the adrenal glands but also address the underlying conditions that are causing the adrenal fatigue in the first place.

In Chapter 11, you read about ways to replace minerals and vitamins, increase cellular energy levels, reduce inflammation, provide antioxidant support, and normalize your body's pH and intestinal health. Chapter 11 also discusses getting better sleep with supplements, using herbs, and undergoing detoxification.

Eating and exercising well

Two big ways that you can help your adrenal glands are committing to a regular exercise regimen and eating the right foods. In Chapter 12, we give you exercise pointers that can help you feel better, reduce stress, and improve your sleep, all of which reduce adrenal stress. An exercise regimen consists of aerobics (like walking and biking), resistance training (such as lifting weights), and meditative exercises (like yoga and t'ai chi).

This chapter also provides some basic nutrition guidelines to improve adrenal health and combat adrenal fatigue. You read about nutritious, high-quality food that not only boosts adrenal gland function but also tastes delicious.

Taking care of yourself at work

Work-related stress is epidemic. Many people spend more time at work than with their families. In Chapter 13, you read about ways to reduce stress, incorporate exercise into your daily routine, and eat healthier in the workplace. We explain the importance of enjoying some time off from work and help you avoid brain fog in the workplace, where you need to be able to think clearly and function well.

Trying Great Recipes for Combatting Adrenal Fatigue

In Part IV, the focus is on getting you in the kitchen for some great, tasty recipes to help combat adrenal fatigue. From energizing breakfasts in Chapter 14 to fuel-food lunches in Chapter 15 to delicious dinners in Chapter 16, you get some of coauthor Wendy Jo's mouthwatering recipes that not only satisfy the palate but also combat adrenal fatigue and help you flourish.

If you're going to sneak in a snack, why not make it healthy and delicious? In Chapter 17, Wendy Jo shares some ideas for snacks and desserts that both fortify and satisfy you.

Chapter 2

Understanding the Basics of Adrenal Gland Function

*I*f you think of your body as an orchestra, the adrenal glands are the conductors. They regulate many important processes:

✔ Producing hormones

✔ Keeping blood pressure, blood chemistry, and the body's acid-base balance in check

✔ Maintaining your strength and vitality, as the adrenal glands work with a number of other parts of the body, especially the hypothalamus and the pituitary gland

✔ Regulating the immune system; if you have adrenal fatigue, then your immune system isn't as effective in fighting off infection

These conductors are responsible for keeping your body in balance in response to the many stresses, both psychological and physical, that you're exposed to on a daily basis. If your adrenal glands are out of kilter, your body slowly begins to wear down. When the adrenal glands aren't healthy, you're unable to cope with daily stresses.

The good news is that if you keep your adrenal glands healthy, the other systems in your body will work that much better. You'll feel better, get a better night's rest, and have more energy and passion in your daily life.

In this chapter, you find out about the adrenal glands' anatomy and functions. When you begin to recognize all that the adrenal glands are responsible for, you'll be able to recognize the early warning signs and symptoms of adrenal fatigue and why they're important.

Checking Out the Anatomy of an Adrenal Gland

Before delving into adrenal fatigue, you should have a working knowledge of the structure and function of the adrenal glands. Understanding where they are and how they interact with other organs of the body is important in helping yourself, because the more you know, the better advocate you can be for your own health.

The two adrenal glands are shaped like little triangles, and they sit atop the kidneys in much the same way a hat sits atop someone's head (see Figure 2-1). Using the spine as a reference, they're under your ribs where your mid back area (the *thoracic spine*) meets your lower back (the *lumbar spine*). Because the adrenal glands and the kidneys are so attached to one another, health conditions that affect the adrenal glands can affect the kidneys as well. In Chinese medicine, the kidneys and adrenal glands are actually thought of as being one organ system.

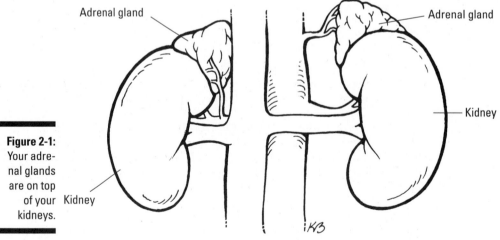

Figure 2-1: Your adrenal glands are on top of your kidneys.

Illustration by Kathryn Born, MA

Each adrenal gland has an outer part and an inner part, all enclosed by a capsule (see Figure 2-2). Here's what each part does:

- **Adrenal capsule:** This capsule of connective tissue encases the adrenal gland, serving as a protective layer. It's primarily composed of adipose tissue (fat).

- **Adrenal cortex:** This outer part of the adrenal gland comprises more than 75 percent of the adrenal gland. It has three zones, each of which performs a distinct function:

  - The *zona glomerulosa* makes the blood-pressure regulating hormone aldosterone.

  - The *zona fasciculata* makes cortisol.

  - The *zona reticularis* makes sex hormones such as dehydroepian-drosterone (commonly known as DHEA).

- **Adrenal medulla:** This inner part of the adrenal gland produces hormones such as epinephrine.

You read about the importance of all these hormones in the next section.

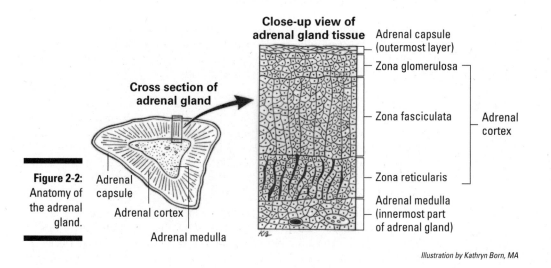

Figure 2-2: Anatomy of the adrenal gland.

Illustration by Kathryn Born, MA

Producing Necessary Hormones

The adrenal glands are *endocrine glands,* which means they secrete stuff inside your body that can affect the functioning and/or the activity level of other organs. You may remember from school that the endocrine system also includes the hypothalamus, pituitary gland, thyroid gland, and reproductive organs, namely the ovaries and testes. Optimal functioning of the adrenal gland is important for the entire endocrine system to work well.

Your adrenal glands help regulate many important biological processes by producing hormones. A *hormone* is a substance, usually a protein, that an organ produces to help regulate or control the function of another organ or body process. For example, the ovaries and the adrenal glands make estrogen, which regulates the menstrual cycle. Another important example of the endocrine system at work is the production of cortisol by the adrenal glands; cortisol production depends on hormones made by the hypothalamus and pituitary gland.

The adrenal glands, as you find out in this section, make aldosterone, cortisol, sex hormones, epinephrine, and norepinephrine.

The word *hormone* comes from the Greek. It means "to set in motion, excite, stimulate."

Analyzing aldosterone

Aldosterone is a hormone produced by the adrenal cortex, specifically the *zona glomerulosa* (for details, see the earlier section "Checking Out the Anatomy of an Adrenal Gland"). Aldosterone is important in regulating blood pressure and regulating salt and water in the body:

- **Regulating blood pressure:** In treating high blood pressure, physicians and other healthcare providers look at the renin-angiotensin-aldosterone system (RAAS). Aldosterone production is closely linked to the kidneys, which make the hormones renin and angiotensin. Angiotensin directly stimulates the adrenal glands to produce aldosterone; aldosterone then regulates blood pressure by causing the kidneys to hold on to more sodium when the blood pressure is low.

  In adrenal fatigue, the adrenal glands may not produce adequate amounts of aldosterone (in addition to not producing other hormones like cortisol). This is a major cause of the low blood pressure that can be seen in adrenal fatigue.

- **Regulating salt and water:** If you consume too much sodium in your diet, the high sodium intake causes a decrease in the production of aldosterone by the adrenal glands, so your kidneys eliminate the excess sodium. If you're dehydrated or your blood pressure is low, your adrenal glands make more aldosterone to signal the kidneys to hold on to that sodium.

Shutting off inflammation

Inflammation is your body's natural response to pathogens (germs) and conditions such as an acute injury or trauma. Acute inflammation helps the body heal from the acute injury, infection, and/or illness. During an acute inflammatory response, the adrenal glands increase cortisol production to help shut off this response when it's no longer needed. This is a normal physiologic process.

On the other hand, *sustained* inflammation (such as in chronic illness) can have very bad effects on the body. In many people's lives, the stress is constant, which causes the adrenal glands to work overtime to produce cortisol. The adrenal glands are trying to do what they were designed to do: make cortisol in response to the increased stress. Over time, overproduction of cortisol can cause damage and increase the risk of heart disease and osteoporosis. Chapter 7 has examples of chronic illnesses and chronic inflammatory conditions that cause the adrenals to produce cortisol constantly.

✔ **Helping the kidneys maintain acid-base balance:** Aldosterone can stimulate the kidneys to eliminate the excess acid the body doesn't need. Adrenal fatigue can affect the kidneys' ability to eliminate this excess acid.

Confronting cortisol

The adrenal glands (specifically, the *zona fasciculata*) produce the hormone cortisol. Cortisol has multiple functions, and every one of them is vital:

✔ Cortisol is important for your immune health because it reduces inflammation (see the nearby sidebar).

✔ Cortisol prevents your blood glucose levels from dropping too low (a condition called *hypoglycemia*).

✔ Cortisol helps regulate blood pressure. The adrenal glands increase cortisol production when your blood pressure is low.

The adrenals produce cortisol 24 hours a day, 7 days a week. In most people, cortisol production increases dramatically at about 4:00 a.m. and is at its highest level around 8:00 a.m. The secretion of cortisol tends to be at its lowest level in the afternoon and at night.

Surveying sexy hormones

The adrenal glands (in particular, the *zona reticularis*) are responsible for producing sex hormones. Examples of these hormones are DHEA, pregnenolone, and androstenedione. The hormones are important in the production of testosterone in the testes and estradiol (think estrogen) in the ovaries, but they also affect other organs.

✔ **DHEA:** DHEA, or dehydroepiandrosterone, helps maintain your immune system. It has a role in lowering inflammation. As you get older, your body produces less DHEA. The adrenal glands' decrease in DHEA production can actually begin in your early thirties. In many chronic illnesses, the levels of DHEA can be very low.

✔ **Pregnenolone:** Pregnenolone is called a *precursor hormone* because it's needed for the production of many other hormones, one of them being DHEA. Normally, pregnenolone blocks the effects of cortisol (see the preceding section). Studies have shown that pregnenolone has beneficial effects on memory and nerve function. It also helps you get a good night's sleep.

In adrenal fatigue, your body produces less pregnenolone because the adrenal glands synthesize more cortisol at the expense of pregnenolone. Trouble again: Pregnenolone belongs to the group of neurosteroids found in high concentrations in certain areas of the brain. Lower pregnenolone levels may help explain symptoms of adrenal fatigue such as poor memory, confusion, and brain fog. You can read more about this in Chapter 4.

✔ **Androstenedione:** This hormone is closely linked to testosterone and estradiol:

• **Testosterone:** Testosterone plays a key role in the development of male reproductive tissues such as the testes and prostate. It's responsible for secondary sexual characteristics such as increased muscle, increased bone mass, and the growth of body hair. Androstenedione (from the adrenal glands) is the common precursor of testosterone.

Testosterone is important for women as well. It helps women improve muscle strength as well as maintain healthy bone mass. It's also vital for maintaining a healthy libido in women.

• **Estradiol:** The adrenal glands produce androstenedione, which is essential for producing estradiol. Estradiol, which is one of the three estrogens occurring in women, is the predominant estrogen during the reproductive years.

If DHEA, pregnenolone, and androstenedione aren't being produced due to adrenal fatigue, the production of estrogen and testosterone can decrease. These two hormones are vital for women's and men's health. An estrogen deficiency in women, for example, can increase the risk of heart disease. A low testosterone level in men is an important cause of fatigue and osteoporosis (yes, osteoporosis does occur in men!).

Examining epinephrine and norepinephrine

Everybody has been really scared at one time or another. Think about a experiencing a near-miss in traffic, finding a rattlesnake on the hiking trail, or hearing your child scream in the front yard. Everything changes instantly.

You may have felt the adrenaline rush as an immediate flow of something from your middle back out to your arms and legs. At that point, your heart rate was rapid. Maybe you felt flushed, broke out in a sweat, or had palpitations. Your blood pressure probably increased. These body changes are due to the hormones *epinephrine,* also called *adrenaline,* and norepinephrine.

If you were a cave dweller, a shot of adrenaline could help you run from a saber-toothed tiger. And in stories about amazing feats of strength — with headlines like "Mother lifts car off baby" — that feat may be due to epinephrine.

Epinephrine and norepinephrine are the two hormones produced in the inner aspect of the adrenal gland — the adrenal medulla. They're big contributors to your body's fight-or-flight response, and they affect the body's nervous system. To give you a little neurologist talk, the *sympathetic nervous system* is activated during a fight-or-flight response, and the *parasympathetic* is activated when the body is relaxed.

In our hectic, stressed-out world, the adrenal glands continually make epinephrine and norepinephrine. Having increased levels of these fight-or-flight hormones in your body is not healthy. Over time, they can contribute to the development of hypertension, heart damage, and kidney disease.

Recognizing the Adrenal Glands' Importance to Blood and pH Balance

The adrenal glands are organs that work many wonders. In addition to regulating blood pressure, these glands work in conjunction with the kidneys to regulate blood chemistry.

The adrenal glands are also vital in maintaining acid-base (pH) balance in the body. In this section, you find out more about the adrenal glands' roles in all this regulation.

Highs and lows: Pondering blood pressure

Blood pressure is the pressure your blood exerts on the walls of your arteries. It's a vital sign and usually one of the first measurements a healthcare provider takes. Most health professionals identify a blood pressure as normal if it's around 120 for the top number and 80 for the bottom number.

Hormones from the adrenals can send your blood pressure way up or way down. Neither extreme is good. In response to a stressor, the hormones produced by the adrenal glands (mainly epinephrine) can raise your blood pressure. Over time, constant stress on the adrenals can eventually affect their ability to produce adequate levels of these hormones necessary for the fight-or-flight response. This is what happens in adrenal fatigue. You can read much more about the measurement of blood pressure and its importance in adrenal fatigue in Chapter 4.

Natural reactions: Looking at blood chemistry

The adrenals are vital in keeping your blood chemistry in a normal range. Three of the most important aspects of your blood chemistry are the sodium, potassium, and blood glucose levels:

- ✔ **Sodium:** The level of sodium in your body is regulated by the adrenal glands and the kidneys. Basically, if you consume too much sodium (salt), the adrenal glands' production of the hormone aldosterone decreases, so the kidneys eliminate the excess sodium.

  People in the United States consume way more sodium than they need. One of the biggest culprits in this regard is processed food, so read your labels! Also reduce the amount of salt you add to your food — ¼ teaspoon table salt is the equivalent of nearly 600 milligrams sodium. In general, the American Heart Association recommends that you take in no more than 2,000 milligrams sodium per day, and less is usually better. Websites like www.nutritiondata.com can be invaluable in providing nutritional information.

- ✔ **Potassium:** As with sodium, the adrenals work in conjunction with the kidneys to regulate the potassium balance in the body. If you eat a meal high in potassium, this signals the adrenal glands to increase the production of aldosterone, which stimulates the kidneys to eliminate excess potassium.

In advanced stages of adrenal fatigue, you may find that the potassium level (as measured in the blood) is higher than normal because of the adrenal glands' overall decrease in aldosterone production.

✔ **Blood glucose:** The adrenals also affect blood glucose (blood sugar) levels in the body. Any state that elevates the production of cortisol is associated with increased blood glucose and can increase the likelihood of developing diabetes. Cortisol can make the body resistant to the actions of insulin, and insulin resistance is a cause of Type II diabetes.

Normal adrenal function tends to produce a healthy body. By contrast, adrenal fatigue can affect the way your body handles sodium, potassium, and blood glucose. See Chapter 4 for details.

A fine line: Handling pH balance

The adrenals work with the kidneys to regulate the acid-base balance (also called pH) in your body. Human blood is supposed to be slightly basic, with a pH of approximately 7.35.

The pH numbers are all about the "power of hydrogen." A low number (acidic) means lots of hydrogen ions, and a high number (basic) means few hydrogen ions. Vinegar has a pH of about 2.4, bleach has a pH of about 12.4, and water is right down the middle at pH 7.0.

Inside the cells of your body, many reactions and enzymes require the right pH to work efficiently. *Acidosis* (excess acid), when unchecked, is a cause of total body inflammation. Ouch!

Did you know that the foods that you eat can be acidic or alkaline? If you eat foods that are very acidic, such as foods high in sugar, you send a signal to the adrenals to increase the production of aldosterone (described earlier in this chapter). This increase then sends a signal to the kidneys to eliminate the excess hydrogen ions in the urine and help the body reach a normal pH. A continued acid load over time can overwork your adrenal glands and your kidneys. Your kidneys won't eliminate the excess acid as well, beginning a vicious cycle of inflammation and worsening, ongoing fatigue.

One initial tipoff that you may have a problem with acidosis is a simple blood test. Healthcare providers routinely order a blood chemistry panel, called either a *CHEM-7* or a *basic metabolic panel.* (These panels amount to seven or eight blood tests at once.) In that panel are a number of electrolyte values, including sodium and potassium, and blood glucose values, along with the bicarbonate level. A normal bicarbonate value is 24 milliequivalents per liter (meq/L) or higher; a level lower than this may be a sign that your blood is too acidic. That being said, further testing (as Chapter 5 describes) is needed to better define the pH of the body.

Interacting with Other Parts of the Body

Your body is a wonderful chemical factory, with endocrine glands making hormones that tell the body what to do. And nothing in the body occurs in isolation. The adrenal glands are essential for other organs in the body to work well.

When healthcare practitioners think about adrenal gland function in the setting of adrenal fatigue, they aren't just thinking about the adrenal glands. They're often thinking about how the adrenal glands work in conjunction with two other organs, namely the hypothalamus and pituitary gland. The interaction of the hormones produced by these three organs is often referred to as the *HPA axis*.

Here's the rundown on the hypothalamus, pituitary gland, and a couple of other organs that act on, interact with, or are affected by the adrenal glands:

- **Hypothalamus:** The hypothalamus is the starter. Located in the brain, it's responsible for producing many hormones that stimulate the release of other hormones in the body. The hypothalamus produces corticotropin-releasing hormone (CRH), which then stimulates the pituitary gland to produce adrenocorticotropic hormone (ACTH); this stimulates the adrenal gland to make cortisol. The adrenal glands can't produce cortisol if the hypothalamus doesn't first produce CRH.

  The hypothalamus is also a great stimulator for the thyroid gland.

- **Pituitary:** The pituitary gland, which is about the size of a pea, sits just under the hypothalamus. The pituitary makes ACTH, which in turn stimulates the production of cortisol in the adrenal glands. As a bonus, the pituitary controls growth, breast milk production, sex organ function, thyroid function, and more.

- **Thyroid:** The major function of the thyroid, which is in your neck, is controlling the body's metabolism. It works in concert with the adrenals. There's a tremendous overlap between adrenal fatigue and thyroid dysfunction. If you jump to Chapter 7, you can read about the interaction between the thyroid and adrenal glands.

- **Kidneys:** The adrenal glands work with the kidneys to help control blood pressure, keep electrolytes in balance, and keep the body in a normal acid-base balance. The kidneys act as the filter of the body; their job consists of excreting all the body's toxins that build up on a daily basis. In addition, they're important in preventing anemia and in keeping bones healthy and strong.

Chapter 3

Defining Adrenal Fatigue

· ·

· ·

Adrenal fatigue is probably one of the most underdiagnosed and under-recognized conditions by physicians and other healthcare providers. Yet there are likely thousands, if not millions, who suffer from this condition. How can you tell if you or someone you know has adrenal fatigue? Having some background information helps. This chapter discusses factors that may lead to adrenal fatigue, lists its stages, and distinguishes between adrenal fatigue and similar syndromes. (Flip to Chapter 4 for the scoop on specific symptoms.)

Focusing on Factors That May Lead to Adrenal Fatigue

At the most basic level, *adrenal fatigue* refers to chronically overworked and overstressed adrenal glands that can become completely exhausted over time. Picture yourself working double shifts for a month straight with little sleep and little opportunity to take a break and recover. You're tired and worn out, right? During the development of adrenal fatigue, the adrenal glands act the same way; they're constantly working hard with little or no chance to rest. Over time, they become unable to do their job effectively.

Adrenal fatigue is an example of organ dysfunction in response to inflammation. Early on, sustained inflammation and illness stimulate the adrenals to produce cortisol. Eventually, the adrenal glands are so fatigued that they aren't able to produce enough of the hormones such as cortisol and aldosterone that the body needs to function on a daily basis. (Chapter 2 goes into detail on adrenal hormones.)

Adrenal fatigue develops in five stages. Before you review these stages (described later in this chapter), consider the following factors, which are important in the development of adrenal fatigue. (Also check out Part II for the full scoop on specific triggers.)

Everyone is different; some people are able to deal with a particular stressor for years before developing adrenal fatigue. For others, a single traumatic event triggers the development of adrenal fatigue. Thus, the time for someone to develop adrenal fatigue differs. That being said, it's often a chronic process that develops over a period of months to years.

Looking at heredity

Some experts hypothesize that some people are born with more adrenal reserve than others — in other words, their adrenal glands have a better constitution, which delays the development of adrenal fatigue. Their adrenal glands seem to be better able to deal with a chronic illness and stress compared to other people's. The support for this idea is anecdotal, based on conversations with other alternative healthcare practitioners.

A 2013 article from the journal *Annals of the New York Academy of Sciences* cites data that supports the idea that some people are genetically susceptible to chronic inflammation. This genetic component may be related to an abnormality in the steroid (cortisol) receptor, more commonly referred to as the glucocorticoid receptor (GR). Abnormalities in the GR may be responsible for the development of certain autoimmune diseases as well as the decrease in cortisol production by the adrenal glands.

The article hypothesizes that abnormalities of the GR not only increase total body inflammation but also impair the actions of the hypothalamic-pituitary-adrenal (HPA) axis and affect the ability of the adrenal glands to produce cortisol. How much an individual is affected by abnormalities in this receptor may determine the degree to which he or she is prone to develop inflammation and chronic illness as well as adrenal fatigue.

Examining early stressors

Health professionals often think of adrenal fatigue as an adult syndrome; however, early stressors may significantly impact cortisol secretion later in life.

A 2011 article from the journal *Endocrinology* examined the relationships among several stress-related disorders, including chronic pain, chronic fatigue, and post-traumatic stress disorder. Despite the significant physical and psychological stress that these syndromes can cause, researchers found very low cortisol levels in the blood. (A typical response to stress is increased cortisol in the blood; cortisol eventually drops back to a normal level after the stress passes.)

The investigators concluded that the younger the age of the person when the stress began, the greater the likelihood of developing lower cortisol levels earlier in life. For someone subjected to repeated stressors at a young age, a type of "developmental programming" may occur: Over time, the repeated stresses cause changes in the body's "software" that permanently decrease the amount of cortisol produced by the adrenal glands.

Children and teenagers are now being diagnosed with inflammatory conditions that were once thought to affect only adults, including diabetes and obesity. Adrenal fatigue is linked to inflammation, so if you had one of these conditions as a child, you may be more likely to develop adrenal fatigue at a younger age.

Making sense of medication effects

Commonly prescribed medications, such as inhaled steroids and statin medications, are likely important in the development of adrenal fatigue.

Steroid medications

Physicians prescribe steroid medication such as prednisone to treat many conditions, from asthma and emphysema to debilitating forms of arthritis and lupus. Physicians know that when someone takes oral steroids for a few days, it decreases the ability of the adrenal glands to produce cortisol. For many chronic conditions, people require multiple doses of oral prednisone. Many studies suggest that chronic use of orally prescribed steroids can affect the adrenal glands' ability to produce cortisol.

Although much attention in the medical community has focused on oral steroids, little attention has focused on the effects of *inhaled* steroids and adrenal fatigue. Given that millions of children and adults are prescribed inhaled steroids to take daily for chronic lung conditions, it's important to understand the effects of long-term inhaled use on adrenal function.

In an article from the journal *Allergy, Asthma, and Clinical Immunology* published in 2010, researchers examined the role of inhaled steroids on the development of *suppression* of adrenal gland function; this means that the adrenal glands' ability to produce cortisol is inhibited. In particular, children who've been on high doses of inhaled steroids for asthma can show effects of adrenal suppression. It's feasible that the adrenal suppression due to the use of inhaled steroids may contribute to adrenal fatigue over time. Inhaled steroids may affect the adrenal glands' ability to produce cortisol when needed, in a similar way that oral steroids do, for up to one year after someone discontinues the inhaled steroids.

Statin medications

Statin medications are a commonly prescribed class of medications in the treatment of high cholesterol and heart disease. Cholesterol is the fundamental ingredient in the synthesis of hormones from the adrenal glands. Statin medications inhibit the synthesis of cholesterol, so could they play a role in the development of adrenal fatigue?

A study in the *Archives of Internal Medicine* in 2012 examined more than 1,000 individuals who were taking a statin medication. The authors looked at two medications, simvastatin (Zocor) and pravastatin (Pravachol). The authors noted that 40 percent of those taking simvastatin reported increased fatigue. Increased fatigue was reported with less frequency with pravastatin.

Was the reported fatigue simply a side effect of the statin medication itself, or did the medication affect the adrenal glands' functioning, causing the fatigue? Two other lab-based studies may shed some light on this question. In a 2003 article from the *British Journal of Pharmacology,* investigators felt that simvastatin decreased the sensitivity of the adrenal glands and decreased the secretion of aldosterone, a major adrenal hormone. A lab-based study from the *Journal of Pharmacology and Experimental Therapeutics* in 2008 noted that simvastatin can inhibit the production of the stress hormones epinephrine and norepinephrine, which are responsible for the fight-or-flight reaction. If you are on a statin medication and are dealing with fatigue, ask your healthcare practitioner whether it would be prudent to discontinue the medication and have your adrenal function evaluated.

Evaluating environmental and psychological factors

Concerning the development of adrenal fatigue, you can't ignore environmental factors or the things that people do to themselves. People drink alcohol to excess, smoke too many cigarettes, and even use drugs such as heroin and cocaine. These activities can fatigue the adrenal glands big time.

Smoking increases the body's inflammatory response dramatically. Cigarettes contain toxins and heavy metals, including cadmium and lead, which are also acute stressors for the adrenals. Cocaine increases the workload of the adrenal glands by pushing them to make higher amounts of epinephrine and norepinephrine. The mega levels of these hormones produced after cocaine ingestion not only stress out the adrenal glands but can also cause dangerously high blood pressures and increase the risk of developing an acute stroke and/or heart attack.

Psychological stressors are just as potent as physical and environmental ones. Adrenal fatigue is associated with depression and post-traumatic stress disorder. An article from *Biological Psychiatry* in February 2013 demonstrated that in someone diagnosed with major depression, not only is the functioning of the adrenal glands altered, but so is the interaction among the hypothalamus, pituitary, and adrenal glands. Abnormal functioning of these glands can produce low levels of cortisol, and this can be a cause of depression. Please refer to Chapter 4 for info concerning the relationship between adrenal fatigue and depression, and see Chapter 18 for ways to beat depression.

Staging Adrenal Fatigue

The development of adrenal fatigue has five phases:

1. **Adrenal surge:** A stimulus causes a rise in the secretion of cortisol and other hormones such as aldosterone, epinephrine, and norepinephrine from the adrenal glands (see Chapter 2 for info on these hormones). This stimulus can be many things, including chronic inflammation and illness.

2. **Sustained adrenal secretion:** The stimulus becomes constant, which causes more sustained cortisol secretion over time.

3. **Turning point stage:** In response to the stimulus, the adrenal glands work overtime to maintain the cortisol secretion. Although they're still able to maintain the necessary levels of cortisol and other adrenal hormones, they're beginning to develop fatigue in this stage.

4. **Adrenal decline:** The adrenal glands begin to tire. They can no longer maintain the high levels of cortisol, and consequently the cortisol levels begin to decline.

5. **Adrenal exhaustion:** The adrenal glands experience utter exhaustion.

The adrenal surge

The first stage involves a dramatic surge in several adrenal hormones when the adrenal glands are stressed. In Part II, you read about many triggers of adrenal fatigue, including illness, infection, stress, and so forth. Many of them can occur at the same time. That's a lot for your adrenals to take!

Sustained hormone secretion

In the face of one or more chronic stressors, the surge of cortisol secretion is constant and persists for a long time. Consequences of this cortisol surge include the following:

- A weakened immune system and susceptibility to infections
- Bone thinning and bone loss, with osteoporosis-type changes

✔ High blood pressure

✔ *Hyperglycemia* (higher-than-normal blood sugars) and *metabolic syndrome* (a constellation of medical conditions including hyperglycemia, high blood pressure, obesity, and high triglycerides); please refer to Chapter 4 for more information on these

Note: Cushing's syndrome, which we discuss later in this chapter, also produces some of these symptoms.

Aldosterone secretion can increase as well. This hormone, which is produced by the adrenal glands' *zona glomerulosa* (see Chapter 2), is important for regulating blood pressure and volume. A consequence of increased aldosterone secretion in this early stage is higher-than-normal blood pressure.

The secretion of the fight-or-flight hormones, epinephrine and norepinephrine, can increase in this stage as well. As with cortisol, the production of these hormones can be sustained in the face of constant stimuli (such as stress). Many people have elevated levels of these fight-or-flight hormones but don't have any symptoms. Some symptoms that may be present include high blood pressure, a fast heart rate, and palpitations.

Note that many other medical conditions can also cause these symptoms. That's why a holistic evaluation by a healthcare provider is important.

 Believe it or not, going to the physician's office can be a cause of adrenal stress. In *white coat hypertension,* a person's blood pressure increases when he or she goes to a physician's office. This condition isn't benign, because a similar surge of adrenal hormones can occur due to other stressors over the course of the day.

The turning point stage

The third stage of adrenal fatigue is the *turning point* stage. Two seemingly opposite things occur:

✔ The adrenal glands are working hard to maintain constant secretion of cortisol and other adrenal hormones.

✔ At the same time, the adrenal glands are beginning to get fatigued; they're starting to become unable to maintain the same level of hormone production as before. The adrenal glands are essentially running out of gas, using a lot of their reserves to keep producing cortisol. People can begin to experience some of the following symptoms:

   • Increased tiredness

   • Hypoglycemia (low blood glucose levels)

- Lower blood pressure
- Dizziness and lightheadedness when standing too quickly

See Chapter 4 for information about these signs and symptoms.

Adrenal decline

The fourth stage of adrenal fatigue concerns a decline in adrenal function. The adrenal glands are unable to keep up with the metabolic demands for increased cortisol, so cortisol secretion begins to decrease. The person in this stage can experience the following signs and symptoms due to the decline in hormonal production:

- ✔ Loss of libido
- ✔ Worsening low blood pressure than in the previous stage
- ✔ Increased dizziness and lightheadedness with standing
- ✔ Increased confusion and problems with thinking
- ✔ Salt cravings

The decline in adrenal function can also intensify the harmful stimulus that started the whole process, as the body is becoming more and more unable to deal with it. In the setting of adrenal decline, if you were to acquire a bacterial infection, for example, you would be more affected by the infection than someone with an intact immune system would. The infection may stay around longer, and you may have more complications as a result of the infection.

Adrenal exhaustion

In the final stage, the adrenal glands are completely wiped out. No more adrenal reserve is left: The adrenal glands have completely run out of gas. Some of the symptoms in this stage are similar to those of Addison's disease, described later in this chapter. The person with adrenal exhaustion can be extremely fatigued all the time and be unable to get out of bed or function normally. He or she can be confused and have significant problems thinking.

The adrenal glands are resilient, and with the right testing and personalized treatment plan, adrenal fatigue can be overcome. The challenge for patients and healthcare professionals is recognizing and treating adrenal fatigue early enough, before it progresses to adrenal exhaustion.

Keeping an Eye on Syndromes That Are Related to Adrenal Fatigue

Patients and healthcare providers alike often confuse other syndromes with adrenal fatigue. Although their features may overlap with adrenal fatigue (involving the production of cortisol and aldosterone), the conditions are in fact quite different. In this section, you read about these syndromes. They include Cushing's syndrome, Addison's disease, and hyperaldosteronism.

Surveying Cushing's syndrome

Cushing's syndrome is a syndrome in which the body produces an excess amount of cortisol, just as in the early stages of adrenal fatigue. Common causes of Cushing's syndrome include the following:

- An *adenoma,* or benign growth on an adrenal gland
- A growth on the pituitary gland that stimulates the production of ACTH (adrenocorticotropic hormone), resulting in excess production of cortisol by the adrenal glands
- Certain cancers, like lung cancer, that can produce ACTH, causing excess cortisol production

Healthcare providers first suspect Cushing's syndrome based on one or more of the following symptoms:

- The presence of a swollen face, which is often referred to as *moon facies*
- A *buffalo hump,* which is a swelling on the back of the neck
- Increased and lower-extremity swelling
- The presence of abdominal obesity, particularly the appearance of abdominal striae (think of *striae* as stretch marks, like in pregnancy)
- One or more aspects of metabolic syndrome, including high blood pressure, high blood glucose levels, obesity, and high triglycerides; *triglycerides* are a form of lipids (like cholesterol) that, when high (as measured on a blood test), can increase the risk of developing heart disease

Unlike adrenal fatigue, the diagnosis of Cushing's can be confirmed by measuring cortisol levels in the urine. Your healthcare provider may ask you to collect your urine in a specialized type of container over a 24-hour period in order to measure the amount of cortisol. A measurement of 50 micrograms of cortisol in 24-hour urine is strongly suggestive of Cushing's syndrome.

The treatment depends on the underlying cause of Cushing's syndrome:

- ✔ If an adrenal adenoma is the cause, the adrenal gland may need to be removed, and you may need adrenal steroid replacement. The same goes for the pituitary gland.

- ✔ If lung cancer is the cause, then the treatment is aimed at the underlying cancer, which can include chemotherapy, radiation therapy, surgery, or a combination of all three.

Analyzing Addison's disease

Adrenal insufficiency, also known as Addison's disease, is an autoimmune condition. Autoimmune diseases like Addison's disease and systemic lupus erythematosus (SLE) occur when the body develops antibodies against itself.

The most common cause of Addison's disease is the production of antibodies that are directed against the adrenal glands. Because of these antibodies, the adrenal glands are unable to produce hormones such as cortisol and aldosterone. Some of the symptoms of this condition overlap with the adrenal decline stage of adrenal fatigue. Here are some key symptoms that can suggest Addison's disease:

- ✔ When this condition first begins, you may experience fatigue, lightheadedness, and *orthostatic hypotension* (a drop in blood pressure when moving from lying down to either a sitting or standing position).

- ✔ Another classic finding is hyperpigmentation. You may see these pigmented areas along the creases of your hands.

- ✔ You may notice decreased hair growth under your armpits or in your pubic area.

- ✔ Key lab findings on blood work can include low sodium levels *(hyponatremia)* and high potassium levels *(hyperkalemia).*

The diagnosis of Addison's disease can be confirmed by blood tests:

- ✔ Your healthcare provider may suspect a diagnosis of Addison's disease if you have a low cortisol level, usually less than 5 milligrams per deciliter in a blood test conducted in the morning.

- ✔ If cortisol is low, then you need a confirming test, namely an adrenal gland challenge called a *cosyntropin stimulation test.* With this test, your healthcare provider measures your baseline cortisol, intravenously injects cosyntropin (a synthetic derivative of ACTH, which is made in the pituitary gland), and measures your cortisol levels 30 and 60 minutes after. A rise of 10 units above the baseline is usually considered an adequate response to ACTH. If this response is present, then Addison's disease is not.

Autoimmune conditions often occur together. If Addison's disease is diagnosed, it's highly probable another autoimmune condition is present. If you're diagnosed with Addison's disease, look for other autoimmune conditions. Examples include Type I diabetes mellitus and hypothyroidism due to Hashimoto's thyroiditis.

The treatment of Addison's disease consists of medications to substitute for both cortisol and aldosterone. They include *hydrocortisone,* which is a synthetic cortisol that's given to help restore blood pressure, given that the adrenal gland is unable to make cortisol.

A dreaded complication of Addison's disease is an *Addisonian crisis.* This occurs in the setting of an acute stressor, such as an infection. The adrenal glands can't make enough cortisol to deal with the stressor. The affected person often presents with very low blood pressure in a condition called *shock.* The treatment involves intravenous steroids, such as hydrocortisone, which can be life-saving. If you've been diagnosed with Addison's disease and you're already on steroid replacement, then this medication needs to be increased during the time of an acute stressor, such as a really bad infection.

Assessing excess aldosterone

In *hyperaldosteronism,* the body produces too much aldosterone (just like in the early stages of adrenal fatigue). The most common cause of this condition is an *adrenal adenoma,* a benign growth on an adrenal gland. Another common cause is *hyperplasia,* a thickening of both adrenal glands.

Symptoms of excess aldosterone production include the following:

✔ High blood pressure that's difficult to control, despite using multiple medications

✔ On blood tests, persistently low potassium *(hypokalemia),* despite a more than adequate potassium replacement

Blood tests can confirm a diagnosis of hyperaldosteronism. Your healthcare provider will order the blood levels of the hormones renin and aldosterone. A very high aldosterone level and a very low renin level is confirmatory for this syndrome. Additional imaging tests, such as a CT scan, can confirm the presence of an adenoma.

Here's the treatment for hyperaldosteronism:

✔ If an adenoma is present, physicians usually recommend that it be surgically removed.

✔ If hyperplasia of the adrenal glands is present, then the treatment is the use of medications that inhibit aldosterone secretion, such as spironolactone (Aldactone).

Chapter 4

Recognizing the Symptoms of Adrenal Fatigue

In this chapter, you get acquainted with the many symptoms of adrenal fatigue. Often, people have more than one presenting symptom. Although the most common presenting symptoms include salt cravings and low blood pressure, other symptoms, such as confusion and depression, can also suggest adrenal fatigue.

Unfortunately, you or your medical practitioner may not recognize the symptoms right away. They may be mistaken for signs of another medical condition altogether. It would be wonderful if one symptom pointed to one disease, but that's rarely true; any condition can point to several afflictions. The only way to diagnose adrenal fatigue is to list your symptoms for your practitioner and undergo testing, which we describe in Chapter 5.

Note that different symptoms can occur at each of the five stages of adrenal fatigue; to review the stages, jump to Chapter 3. Part II has details on the major triggers of adrenal fatigue.

Viewing the Vital Signs

When you go to the doctor, typically the first thing the medical technician does is obtain your vital signs, including your temperature, blood pressure, and pulse. Vital signs are a simple way to assess basic body functions. In most cases of adrenal fatigue, these signs are on the low side, but some may be high. This section gives you the scoop on adrenal fatigue symptoms related to your vital signs.

If you begin a treatment plan for adrenal fatigue, keep a written record of all your vital signs, especially your temperature and blood pressure. Don't forget to bring the record with you when you see your healthcare practitioner.

Taking your temperature

A lower-than-normal body temperature can be a sign of adrenal fatigue, especially in the latter stages of adrenal fatigue. Know what your normal body temperature is. For most people, their normal temperature is about 98 degrees Fahrenheit (36.7 degrees Celsius). For some people, the normal baseline body temperature is lower. Some may notice a minor decrease in their normal body temperature over time.

Don't panic. "Normal" body temperature varies a bit, depending on where you take your temperature and even the time of day. Although the most accurate way to obtain an accurate temperature is with a rectal thermometer, a thermometer under the tongue is usually more practical. Think about buying a good thermometer; it's not expensive.

If you notice that your body temperature is lower than normal, take your temperature on a regular basis, at least three times a week, and record the results. If you've begun a treatment program for adrenal fatigue, early on you want to measure your body temperature at least twice a week.

Besides adrenal fatigue, other causes of lower-than-normal body temperature include hypothyroidism (which can slow down your body's metabolism), kidney disease, and acute infection. If you find that your body temperature has dropped to an unusually low level, see your doctor immediately.

Measuring your blood pressure

One of the most common initial symptoms of adrenal fatigue is changes in your blood pressure. You may notice increased dizziness and lightheadedness when you sit up or stand up. In this section, you read about the importance of blood pressure as it relates to adrenal fatigue.

Your blood pressure is made up of two readings — systolic (the upper number) and diastolic (the lower number). It's measured in units of millimeters of mercury (mm Hg), which goes back to the old days when blood pressure was displayed in two thin glass tubes filled with mercury. Normal blood pressure is usually cited as 120/80 ("120 over 80"), and many doctors would love to have everyone close to these numbers.

Taking your blood pressure at home

Depending on your stage of adrenal fatigue and your presenting symptoms, managing your condition may involve measuring your blood pressure at home. With these measurements, you and your healthcare provider can get a better sense of how you're doing day-to-day. Many low-cost blood pressure monitors are available for home use; you can ask your pharmacist or healthcare practitioner for guidance in choosing one.

You measure your blood pressure with a blood pressure cuff (to impress your friends, call it a *sphygmomanometer*). In our experience, you get the most reliable results from devices that use an arm cuff. You strap the cuff on your upper arm and squeeze a bulb to pump it up, or if you're using a digital model, you push a button and the cuff inflates automatically. Then wait for the readings. The digital models give you easy-to-read numbers.

Measure your blood pressure lying, sitting, and standing if you're able. At the very least, try to measure your blood pressure when going from a sitting position to a standing position. To obtain an accurate blood pressure reading, you should maintain each position for at least 90 seconds before checking your blood pressure. For example, after you change from a sitting position to a standing position, stand for at least 90 seconds (if you can) before taking a blood pressure measurement. If you're symptomatic when you stand (that is, lightheaded or dizzy), take your blood pressure sooner, or better yet, have a family member or significant other take your blood pressure if possible. If you feel like you're going to faint, sit down! If you're feeling that lightheaded or dizzy when standing, this is a very strong indication that you need treatment.

Your healthcare provider will likely instruct you to measure your blood pressure on a regular basis, a least once each day. I (coauthor Rich) ask patients to measure their blood pressure at various times during the day. For example, to keep it simple, I may ask them to measure their blood pressure in the morning when they wake up and before dinner. I may ask them to measure their blood pressure before lunch and before they go to sleep the next day. Doing measurements this way helps you pinpoint the point in the day when you're having problems with blood pressure.

Raising your blood pressure

In the early stages of adrenal fatigue, adrenal hormones can elevate your blood pressure. High blood pressure is called *hypertension*. Most physicians define hypertension as a blood pressure above 140/90 mm Hg (a systolic blood pressure above 140 or diastolic blood pressure above 90). It's no secret that stress, illness, and inflammation can elevate blood pressure, and a significant contributor is the increased production of the adrenal hormones cortisol, epinephrine, norepinephrine, and especially aldosterone (see Chapter 2 for details on these hormones).

In day-to-day life, undiagnosed, untreated high blood pressure has earned the name "the silent killer." It increases the risk of heart attack and stroke.

Having low blood pressure

When adrenal fatigue begins to become adrenal burnout, you can develop low blood pressure (technically called *hypotension*), even when you're lying down. Over time, as your adrenal glands are further fatigued, you see a gradual lowering of your baseline blood pressure. In the last stage of adrenal fatigue, which is adrenal exhaustion, blood pressure can be very low because the adrenals aren't producing enough of the hormones cortisol and aldosterone to maintain the blood pressure.

A strict definition of low blood pressure is a value less than 120/80 mm Hg. That being said, everyone's "normal" is different. Some people's baseline blood pressure is as low as 90/40 mm Hg; that's their normal, and they feel fine and dandy with that blood pressure. For others, their blood pressure is often higher. The point is to understand what your normal is and to look for changes from that normal.

Getting dizzy when you stand up

Orthostatic hypotension, or feeling dizzy when you stand up, is one of the commonest symptoms of adrenal fatigue. This symptom often occurs in advanced stages of adrenal fatigue, when the adrenal glands are unable to produce more aldosterone and cortisol, which you need in order to regulate your blood pressure when you sit up or try to stand. Decreased blood flow to the noggin (as we doctors call it) is why you can feel lightheaded or dizzy when you change from one position to another.

Here's how it works: When you change from a lying position to a sitting or standing position, your body has built-in regulatory mechanisms to make sure the blood flow gets to your brain. The adrenal glands increase production of cortisol, aldosterone, epinephrine, and norepinephrine. These hormones increase the activity of your nervous system (specifically, your autonomic nervous system) to try to raise your blood pressure. When your adrenal glands are really worn out, they can't increase the production of these hormones, so you have a blood-flow problem and a nervous-system problem. No wonder you feel dizzy!

When you go to your healthcare provider, begin by telling him or her about any dizziness. Then the practitioner should measure your blood pressure while you're lying down, sitting, and standing.

When your blood pressure is taken in the healthcare practitioner's office, you get only one measurement. To get a fuller picture, measure your blood pressure at home. Please refer to the earlier sidebar "Taking your blood pressure at home."

Your healthcare provider may strongly suspect adrenal fatigue if your blood pressure doesn't increase when you stand up or if it decreases. A systolic blood pressure that doesn't increase by 10 mm Hg upon standing can strongly indicate adrenal fatigue. This is called *Ragland's sign* (see the nearby sidebar "Let's get physical: Reading specific signs of adrenal fatigue").

An official diagnosis of orthostatic hypotension is made when the following are true:

- Your systolic blood pressure (top number) drops 20 mm Hg or more when you go to an upright position.

- Your diastolic blood pressure (bottom number) drops 10 mm Hg or more when you go to an upright position.

- Your heart rate increases when you go to an upright position.

- You're symptomatic (dizzy or lightheaded) when standing up.

Let's get physical: Reading specific signs of adrenal fatigue

Many general symptoms are associated with adrenal fatigue, but here are some very specific signs of the condition:

- **Dizziness when standing:** One symptom is *Ragland's sign.* Normally, when you stand up, your blood pressure rises to accommodate the change in position. If your blood pressure doesn't increase when you stand or if your blood pressure decreases, that's a strong sign that you have adrenal fatigue.

- **Back pain:** Another common sign is *Rogoff's sign,* named after the physician who discovered it. This sign amounts to pain in the mid-back, where the ribs are. The pain may come and go. The pain can be very similar to the pain of a kidney infection or a pulled muscle or a strained ligament, and it can even be confused with pain due to gallbladder inflammation.

Unlike the pain of a pulled muscle, which is self-limited or may go away after a trial of rest and anti-inflammatory medication, the back pain associated with adrenal fatigue pain seems to persist. If you're experiencing this pain and it's not going away (or it keeps coming back), you likely need evaluation for adrenal fatigue.

- **Unreactive pupils:** The third sign comes from a *pupillary test.* Basically, a healthcare provider briefly swings a small flashlight in front of a person's eye. If the pupil fails to constrict and narrow, that can be a sign of adrenal fatigue.

Surveying Blood Sugar

Blood sugar level isn't a vital sign, but it is an important value that needs to be evaluated. Changes in blood sugar levels can be a symptom of adrenal fatigue. In early stages of adrenal fatigue, you may see *hyperglycemia* (high blood sugar). In advanced stages of adrenal fatigue, *hypoglycemia* (low blood sugar) is a common occurrence.

Technically speaking, the blood sugar level is the *blood glucose level. Glucose,* which is a simple sugar present in human blood, is the main source of energy for the body's cells. It's also vital for brain function.

Be aware that many people with adrenal fatigue present with normal blood pressure and blood glucose levels. These are just important things to be aware of concerning signs and symptoms of adrenal fatigue.

Developing high blood sugar: Hyperglycemia

In response to an initial stress, the adrenal glands secrete hormones, including cortisol, epinephrine, and norepinephrine (see Chapter 2). These hormones can raise the blood glucose levels in the body.

What exactly is a normal blood glucose level? Well, if you ever look at the blood work (the "labs") that your healthcare provider orders, a numerical value for a normal blood glucose level is about 70 to 100 milligrams per deciliter (mg/dL). If your blood glucose level is higher than 100 mg/dL, you have *hyperglycemia.* An abnormally high blood glucose level increases the risk of developing other chronic conditions, including diabetes and metabolic syndrome. *Metabolic syndrome* is a syndrome that includes high blood pressure, higher than normal glucose levels, high triglyceride levels, and obesity, among others symptoms. Sustained cortisol secretion over time is a major contributor to the development of the metabolic syndrome.

If your fasting blood glucose level is slightly above normal range (say, approximately 110 to 125 mg/dL), you usually have no symptoms. Just the same, having your blood chemistry tested is important. Having a fasting blood glucose level greater than 126 mg/dL indicates diabetes.

Adrenal fatigue in and of itself usually doesn't cause diabetes; however, for someone with a genetic susceptibility to diabetes, adrenal fatigue — which develops in the setting of increased adrenal hormone production and chronic stress and inflammation — may contribute to the development of diabetes. For someone already diagnosed with diabetes, adrenal fatigue may aggravate diabetes and cause higher-than-normal blood glucose levels.

Handling low blood sugar: Hypoglycemia

Hypoglycemia, or low blood sugar, is related to the action (or lack thereof) of the adrenal hormones cortisol, epinephrine, and norepinephrine. These hormones are called the *counter-regulatory hormones* because they can cause a rise in blood glucose levels. The lack of production of these hormones in the setting of advanced adrenal fatigue is one aspect of what causes hypoglycemia.

The other hormone involved in the genesis of hypoglycemia is insulin, which is made by the pancreas. Insulin secretion increases in the setting of a high-carbohydrate meal. Insulin promotes glucose entry into the cells and thus lowers blood glucose levels. The combination of increased insulin secretion and lack of production of the counter-regulatory hormones contributes to the development of hypoglycemia.

In the setting of advanced adrenal fatigue, hypoglycemia may occur after meals *(postprandial hypoglycemia)* or between meals *(fasting hypoglycemia).*

The symptoms of hypoglycemia can include one or more of the following. (Note that these severe symptoms are very rare in adrenal fatigue. We include them because they may occur, so you should be aware of the symptoms.)

✔ Dizziness or lightheadedness; if your blood glucose levels are really low, you may faint

✔ Lethargy and confusion

✔ Profound sweating

✔ Palpitations (a strange heart rate) or tachycardia (a fast heart rate)

✔ Personality changes; in the phenomenon known as *hypoglycemia unawareness,* the person has noticeable personality changes from his or her baseline but doesn't demonstrate any other symptoms

Do you know anyone who gets cranky around mealtimes? It's amazing how people who want to start arguments on an empty stomach are a lot nicer after they eat. The personality change may be due to low blood sugar. Fortunately, Part IV is devoted to preparing and eating good food. In particular, when you eat a healthy breakfast, you're less likely to bite someone's head off before lunch.

If you have diabetes, you may be especially susceptible to *labile* blood glucose levels (irregular and unpredictable swings in blood glucose). Diabetes is a major stressor of the adrenal glands, so monitor your blood glucose levels closely. See the nearby sidebar for tips on checking your glucose levels.

Checking your blood glucose at home

Your healthcare provider may ask you to monitor your blood glucose levels at home. If you have diabetes, taking these measurements is probably second nature to you. If not, you need to learn the process, which is inexpensive and easy.

You measure your blood glucose levels using a *blood glucose meter* (everybody calls this a *Glucometer*, which is actually a trademark for Bayer's meters). You put a test strip in the meter. Then you put a tiny needle (a lancet) in a spring-loaded lancet device, hold it against your fingertip, and press the button. The lancet makes a tiny puncture, and one drop of blood comes out. Touch the drop with the test strip, and the meter goes to work.

Your healthcare provider can tell you how often to check your blood glucose level. If your blood glucose levels are really labile (up and down), he or she may instruct you to check up to four times a day — often before meals. If you have post-prandial hypoglycemia, then you may need to check the blood glucose level 2 hours after each meal.

Investigating Salt Issues

Adrenal fatigue and issues with sodium and salt are very closely intertwined. In this section, you read about two common salt-related symptoms of adrenal fatigue: edema (swelling) and craving salt.

Swelling up

If you wake up in the morning and notice swelling, especially in your legs, the swelling may be due to adrenal fatigue. Increased cortisol and aldosterone from the adrenal glands can cause your body to retain salt and water, causing you to swell up. The term health professionals use to describe swelling, especially in the legs, is *edema*. Edema is often seen in the later stages of adrenal fatigue.

Some people develop swelling and edema around their abdominal area, without swelling in their extremities; these folks may have difficulty buttoning their shirts. Other clues include shoes or pants that are difficult to put on or that don't fit one day but fit the next. One way doctors evaluate for edema is by pressing around the shin. If the depression exists for some time, you have *pitting*, which is a sign of edema.

If you're suffering from edema, be aware that medical conditions besides adrenal fatigue can cause swelling. They include heart disease and congestive heart failure, kidney disease, and liver disease. A problem with the blood flow in the veins of your legs — called *venous insufficiency* — can also cause swelling. Your healthcare provider will want to further evaluate you for these conditions.

If you have edema, it's important to weigh yourself daily. Changes in fluid weight, or edema weight, can occur on a daily basis. As adrenal fatigue is treated, you may notice a decrease in edema and a related decrease in weight.

Craving salt

One common symptom of adrenal fatigue is continually craving salt. This often happens in the advanced stages of adrenal fatigue. As your adrenal glands become unable to produce enough of the hormone aldosterone, something strange takes place. Aldosterone is responsible for telling the kidneys to retain the salt that your body needs. If your adrenal glands don't produce enough aldosterone, your kidneys eliminate the salt through the urine, leading you to crave more salt.

When aldosterone levels are low, your kidneys aren't fully able to eliminate potassium. While the sodium level in your body is lower than normal, the potassium level may be very high. Too high of a potassium level can affect the heart, slowing it down. Very high potassium levels are potentially fatal.

If you crave salt constantly, drink water to avoid dehydration. Other electrolytes and minerals can be affected in advanced stages of adrenal fatigue as well. Be aware of the potassium content of what you consume. Your healthcare provider may order lab tests (blood work) to follow your sodium and potassium levels.

In the case of adrenal fatigue, your craving for salt is an important symptom. Having too little sodium in your system isn't good. If you're craving salt, your blood pressure may be low; we discuss low blood pressure earlier in this chapter. Chapter 10 discusses salt supplementation.

Feeling Sick and Tired

Many people with adrenal fatigue suffer from a multitude of problems that affect how they feel, their stamina, their sex life, and their ability to fight off infections. You may feel sick, or you may feel tired. Problems can include the following:

- Constant fatigue and weakness
- Difficulty sleeping
- Decreased libido
- Susceptibility to infections
- Recurrent allergies

Healthcare practitioners find that many of these symptoms occur together.

You and your healthcare provider need look at your symptoms in *totality*. If you don't, you may find that you're treating each individual symptom but you're missing the big picture of what's causing your symptoms in the first place.

Being tired all the time

Being constantly tired is one of the hallmark symptoms of adrenal fatigue — *fatigue* is right in the name, after all. A *constant fatigue* doesn't go away. You can try taking afternoon naps or taking vitamins, but nothing seems to help. This fatigue is a consequence of the constant depletion of the reserves of the adrenal glands.

Your degree of tiredness and weakness depends on your baseline body constitution and your stage of adrenal fatigue. Some people can deal with chronic stress for a long period of time and then become exhausted all at once. Others experience a gradual onset and worsening of fatigue. If you're experiencing constant fatigue, seek the help of a qualified medical professional. You may be at risk for adrenal exhaustion.

Having trouble sleeping

You'd think that if you're tired, you'd have little or no trouble hitting the sack and getting a good night's sleep. Think again. Not only does someone with adrenal fatigue not sleep well, but he or she often suffers from *insomnia,* an inability to fall asleep or to stay asleep. Sleeping during the day doesn't help much, either.

One possible reason for difficulty sleeping is sustained and increased cortisol production by the adrenal glands. Here's the medical perspective: At night, when you go to sleep, the production of cortisol usually drops until around 4:00 or 5:00 a.m., when you typically experience a rise in cortisol levels. But sustained cortisol production alters the circadian rhythm of someone with adrenal fatigue. The cortisol revs up the body at night, which is the wrong thing when you want to go to sleep.

In addition to cortisol, the other stress hormones, including epinephrine and norepinephrine, may be produced in higher amounts than normal. So although you may try to get a good night's sleep, the process can be plenty difficult. For details on the effects of adrenal fatigue and sleeping difficulties, jump to Chapter 6.

Losing your sex drive

A decrease or loss of your desire to have sex can be an initial clue that you have adrenal fatigue. When the adrenal glands are making more cortisol in the setting of chronic stress, they may not be making as much testosterone and other sex hormones. Decreased levels of the sex hormones for men and women can cause not only a loss of interest in sex but also a problem with sexual performance.

When faced with this condition, men tend to ask their doctors for prescriptions for medications such as Viagra and Cialis. When adrenal fatigue is present, these medications may have little effect; although they may help with problems with erectile dysfunction, they don't improve libido.

Treatment involves measuring your sex hormone levels (see Chapter 5) and identifying and treating the stressor.

Battling recurrent infections

Have you ever noticed that when you're stressed, you never seem to be infection-free? You're always fighting off some bug, only to catch another one. Adrenal fatigue compromises your immune system, and battling infections such as the following becomes more and more difficult for your body:

- ✔ One of the most common presenting symptoms of adrenal fatigue is recurring lung infections, especially bronchitis. With sustained secretion of cortisol from the adrenal glands, your immune system can't mount an effective immune response.

- ✔ Another common symptom related to adrenal gland function is any infection that seems to take forever to go away. Maybe you acquired a viral illness. With an intact immune system, you should be able to fight off the infection and begin to feel better. With adrenal fatigue, recovery can take a long time.

Too much medication can complicate the problem. Think about what typically happens when you have a bout of acute bronchitis or another infection. You go to your healthcare provider, who may prescribe an antibiotic, which doesn't work if you have a viral illness. If you have recurrent symptoms, you may be prescribed more than one round of antibiotics. Trouble is, not only can frequent antibiotic use alter your intestinal flora (your gut bugs) and make you more susceptible to infection, but it can also promote the overgrowth of the yeast *Candida,* which further alters your immune system. (You can read about the effects of an altered intestinal tract in Chapter 8.)

Furthermore, the more medications you're on, the greater the possibilities of your developing side effects (the so-called *drug-drug interaction*) that can further stress the adrenal glands and further weaken you.

Lyme disease and other chronic infections can be a cause of adrenal fatigue in the first place. Having a comprehensive evaluation done is important not only to confirm the diagnosis of adrenal fatigue but also to search for underlying causes. (Flip to Chapter 5 for the full scoop on testing.)

Dealing with recurring allergies

People with adrenal fatigue tend to have recurrent allergies. These could be food, mold, or seasonal allergies. You may find yourself having more episodes of sneezing, eyes tearing, and coughing.

Allergies can trigger the development of asthma. Fortunately, several studies have pointed out that using probiotics can help alleviate asthma and allergy symptoms. Check out Chapter 11 for details on probiotics.

Irritating Your Bowel and Bladder

Some conditions that affect the bowel and bladder are strongly associated with adrenal fatigue. This section talks about two such medical states: irritable bowel syndrome and interstitial cystitis.

The bowel

You may have noticed that you're not digesting food well. Maybe no matter what you eat, you experience heartburn. Or you're always running to the bathroom due to diarrhea. Or you begin to find yourself straining and suffering from extreme constipation. Maybe certain foods you eat cause you to develop crampy abdominal pain. Maybe the pain comes on even when you're not eating. If you have any or all of the preceding symptoms, you may be experiencing *irritable bowel syndrome* (IBS).

When coauthor Rich was in medical school, the thinking about IBS was that it was purely psychological (that is, severe stress seemed to be the trigger for development of IBS). Minimizing or eliminating the stressor seemed to help the abdominal symptoms. IBS was also considered a diagnosis of exclusion by most medical professionals, meaning that if other causes of *colitis* — inflammation of the large intestine — weren't found either via colonoscopy or endoscopy, the doc was left with the diagnosis of IBS.

That was then; this is now. We're here to tell you that IBS is much more than a psychological stressor. In Chapter 8, you read about how stress and nutrient deficiencies can change the makeup of the bowel flora and about the significant consequences of that change.

The bottom line is this: If you have symptoms of IBS, relay them to your healthcare practitioner. And if you've been diagnosed with IBS, speak with him or her about being evaluated for adrenal fatigue.

The bladder

With adrenal fatigue, a common condition affecting the bladder is *interstitial cystitis* (IC). In plain English, that's *bladder pain syndrome* (BPS). If someone is suffering from IC, adrenal fatigue is likely present and has likely been so for a while.

For many people, especially women in their 30s and 40s, IC is a painful and debilitating condition. The symptoms can include the following:

- Urinary urgency (feeling like you have to go to the bathroom all the time, even when you don't)
- Urinary frequency (frequent voiding)
- *Dysuria,* or a burning sensation when you urinate; the pain of IC can be intense, sharp and knifelike in the bladder
- *Hematuria,* or the presence of blood in the urine
- Back pain and fever

Like adrenal fatigue, interstitial cystitis may not be recognized right away by your healthcare provider. All the preceding symptoms can also indicate a simple urinary tract infection (UTI). If you see your healthcare provider with these complaints, the typical kneejerk reaction is to prescribe an antibiotic for a presumed UTI. A UTI differs from IC in two basic ways:

- IC generally doesn't get better with antibiotics, whereas a UTI does.
- In the case of IC, a culture of the urine is often negative; it doesn't show that an infection is present.

The causes of IC are many, but a major one is food sensitivities, especially sensitivity to gluten. There's a big connection between celiac disease and the development of IC. Foods such as tomatoes can irritate the bladder, too.

A urologist can confirm IC with a *cystoscopy.* With this diagnostic study, a flexible catheter called a *cystoscope* (a bladder cam) enters your bladder so the urologist can look for signs of inflammation.

The treatment for IC is multifaceted and includes keeping a food diary and eliminating gluten from the diet. Being tested for food sensitivities may be helpful. Also, the prescription medication pentosan polysulfate (Elmiron) has helped people with IC. This med is the only oral medication approved by the U.S. FDA for treating interstitial cystitis.

Managing the Mental and the Emotional: Brain Fog and Depression

Some people who have adrenal fatigue present with minimal physical complaints. For them, the initial hint that adrenal fatigue is present is *confusion*, especially brain fog. Don't ignore the mental and emotional effects of adrenal fatigue, which we describe next.

Battling brain fog

Brain fog is a symptom that can occur early in the course of adrenal fatigue. Technically, the field of medicine calls this condition *clouding of consciousness*. With brain fog, you may experience the following:

✔ An inability to concentrate on simple tasks

✔ Problems with short-term memory

✔ Misplacing things and having trouble finding them

✔ Forgetting something that someone just told you

Brain fog can be a big problem at work; your productivity is likely to be dramatically affected.

People with brain fog often wonder if they're experiencing early onset dementia. Probably not. Be aware that brain fog affects short-term memory; your ability to remember your mother's birthday shouldn't be affected. Dementia is a process that occurs over time; brain fog is more of an acute process that occurs over a shorter period of time.

Brain fog is the combined effect of increased cortisol levels, sustained inflammation, and decreased sleep quality and quantity. In other words, adrenal fatigue is a cause of brain fog.

Dealing with depression

Depression, a state of low mood, can be an initial indication that adrenal fatigue is present. Hormonal imbalances have a direct effect on mood. The decrease in adrenal hormone production, especially the sex hormones, can be a direct cause of depression in adrenal fatigue.

Here are some signs and symptoms that can indicate depression:

✔ You lack interest in daily activities.

✔ You eat a lot or hardly eat at all.

✔ You sleep many hours of the day or suffer from insomnia. If the depression is related to adrenal fatigue, insomnia is more likely. Poor sleep due to adrenal fatigue can also contribute to the development of depression.

✔ You gain or lose weight. Concerning depression as it relates to adrenal fatigue, weight gain is more common. The increased production of cortisol can cause weight gain, especially the deposition of belly fat on the anterior aspect of the abdomen (the belly).

Treating your depression is a lot more involved than getting a prescription. If you've been diagnosed with depression, you need a comprehensive and personalized evaluation to look for nutrient deficiencies, anemia, hormonal imbalances, and organ dysfunction (including dysfunction of the adrenal glands, liver, thyroid, and/or kidneys) that can contribute to the development of depression.

Checking Out Other Related Conditions

Other conditions associated with adrenal fatigue include restless legs syndrome and osteoporosis. We cover them here.

Wanting to dance: Restless legs syndrome

Restless legs syndrome (RLS) is a condition in which you experience numbness and tingling in your legs and feel like your legs want to move all the time. The symptoms of RLS can occur especially at night when you want to go to sleep. Moving the legs may help lessen the pain and pins-and-needles sensation in the legs. A patient once said RLS made his legs feel like they wanted to dance, even when he was sitting down.

RLS and adrenal fatigue are closely associated, likely because of hormonal imbalances that link these two conditions. Note that certain nutrient deficiencies have also been implicated in RLS. If you have RLS, your healthcare provider should test you for iron and other nutrient deficiencies, advanced kidney disease, and sleep apnea.

The treatment for RLS includes exercising and avoiding certain stimulants, such as caffeine. The doc may prescribe certain medications, including ropinirole (Requip), to help you manage the symptoms of RLS.

Bad to the bone: Osteoporosis

Osteoporosis (from the Greek, meaning "porous bones") is a decrease in bone density. It commonly occurs in women in their late 40s or early 50s. Osteoporosis has been traditionally associated with postmenopausal women and older men with low testosterone levels. Certain medications and alcohol use can also increase the risk of developing osteoporosis.

That being said, adrenal fatigue is probably an underdiagnosed cause of osteoporosis. Over time, the excess cortisol produced by the adrenal glands can completely demineralize the bone. Decreased sex hormone production also contributes to the development of osteoporosis.

Don't ignore the role of inflammation in osteoporosis. There's a complex interplay between hormonal loss and increased inflammation. A study from *Nutrition Reviews* in 2007 looked at the connection between osteoporosis and inflammation. In menopause, estrogen production decreases. Loss of estrogen was associated with the increased production of protein promoters of the inflammation process. These proteins are called *pro-inflammatory cytokines,* and over time, they can have a damaging effect on bone health.

Your healthcare provider diagnoses osteoporosis by looking for obvious risk factors. He or she can also order a dual-energy X-ray absorptiometry (DEXA) scan. This scan is scored using a *T-score,* which compares a patient's bone density to the peak bone density of a 30-year-old male or female, depending on the sex of the patient.

If you may have osteoporosis, your provider should do a thorough analysis, testing you for adrenal function (and its impairment) and thyroid function. You may need other testing for hormonal imbalances. Depending on the nature of the hormone imbalance, testing for a low testosterone level and simply replacing the testosterone may not be enough, especially in males.

Here are some things you can do to strengthen your bones:

- ✔ Increase physical activity, especially muscle resistance training to increase muscle strength and endurance.

- ✔ Stop tobacco and alcohol use.

- ✔ Take vitamin D supplements, which requires knowing your vitamin D level (see Chapter 11 for details).

- ✔ Increase your calcium and other trace minerals.

It's important to increase your calcium intake but maybe not with the type of supplements you've been taking. Studies show that certain types of calcium supplements may pose a risk to your heart. Increasing your intake of vegetables high in calcium is very helpful. You can read more about this in Chapter 11.

Chapter 5

Testing for Adrenal Fatigue

Could you have adrenal fatigue? In this chapter, you complete a questionnaire to figure out your chances of having adrenal fatigue, and you get the scoop on tests that healthcare professionals use to diagnose or assess risk factors for this condition. (For info on working with these professionals, jump to Chapter 9.)

Maybe your healthcare provider doesn't do all these tests. Remember, you must be the first and best advocate for such testing. Your healthcare provider may change his or her mind, or you may need to search for an additional provider with a focus on alternative medicine.

The cost of many of the specialized tests in this chapter (for example, hair and saliva testing) will likely come out of your pocket. Although we believe much can be gained from testing, finances are a real issue, and your practitioner must understand what you can't do. That's vital in forming a personalized treatment plan.

Filling Out an Adrenal Fatigue Questionnaire

In medical school, I (coauthor Rich) was taught that a healthcare practitioner should be able to diagnose a medical condition just from information obtained from a comprehensive interview (called the *history*) and a thorough physical examination (the *physical*). That was true then, and it's still true now. Virtually everyone in medicine follows this process.

On your initial visit to any healthcare professional (whether conventional medicine or alternative medicine), you fill out a questionnaire about your health history. Together, the history and physical form the basis for an initial diagnosis. In this section, you complete a questionnaire about your medical history. The format is very similar to the one I'd use if I were interviewing you myself.

The goal of the questionnaire is to obtain as much medical information as possible. You and your practitioner need the information not just to confirm the diagnosis but also to evaluate for possible risk factors that contribute to the development of adrenal fatigue. The diagnosis of adrenal fatigue is "new science" and in many ways is a bit of an art form. Adrenal fatigue has many risk factors, but the right healthcare professional is trained to determine whether you have adrenal fatigue after assessing your risk factors and lifestyle and to determine how to proceed.

Walking through the sections

For each section of this questionnaire, please check Yes or No next to each question where applicable. A few questions require you to fill in an answer. After you complete the questionnaire, you tally up your answers to calculate your Adrenal Fatigue Score.

Medical history

In this section, you report common health conditions associated with the development of adrenal fatigue.

1. Do you have a history of any of the following?

Allergies	❏ Yes	❏ No
Anemia	❏ Yes	❏ No
Asthma	❏ Yes	❏ No
Chronic bronchitis	❏ Yes	❏ No
Chronic and recurring respiratory infections (beginning in adulthood)	❏ Yes	❏ No
Cystic fibrosis	❏ Yes	❏ No
Depression	❏ Yes	❏ No
Diabetes	❏ Yes	❏ No
Dialysis	❏ Yes	❏ No
Emphysema	❏ Yes	❏ No
Fibromyalgia	❏ Yes	❏ No
Hypothyroidism	❏ Yes	❏ No
Inflammatory bowel disease	❏ Yes	❏ No
Interstitial cystitis	❏ Yes	❏ No

Irritable bowel syndrome ❏ Yes ❏ No
Kidney disease ❏ Yes ❏ No
Liver disease ❏ Yes ❏ No

2. Have you ever been hospitalized for any of the preceding conditions?

❏ Yes ❏ No

If so, how many times have you been hospitalized? _____

3. Have you ever been told that you have high levels of inflammation?

❏ Yes ❏ No

Surgical history

Surgery can be a cause of acute adrenal gland stress. This section asks you questions about your surgical history.

4. How many surgeries have you had? _____

5. Have you had your adrenal glands removed?

❏ Yes ❏ No

Medications

The use of certain medications, particularly steroids, can be a direct contributor to the development of adrenal fatigue. In this section, you're asked about medication use.

6. Have you ever been on oral steroids?

❏ Yes ❏ No

7. How many times have you been prescribed steroid medication? _____

8. Do you use or have you ever used a steroid inhaler?

❏ Yes ❏ No

9. Have you ever received steroids intravenously?

❏ Yes ❏ No

10. Have you ever taken narcotics/pain medications?

❏ Yes ❏ No

If so, how many years have you been taking pain medication?

_____ months/years

11. Do you take statin medications?

❏ Yes ❏ No

Social history

This section asks about the use of certain substances that directly increase adrenal stress.

12. Do you smoke cigarettes?

    ❑ Yes   ❑ No

    If so, how many cigarettes a day do you smoke? _____

13. Do you drink alcohol?

    ❑ Yes   ❑ No

    If so, how much alcohol do you drink a day? _____

14. Do you take any drugs?

    ❑ Yes   ❑ No

Family history

A history of adrenal fatigue may be an important risk factor for the development of adrenal fatigue. In this section, you answer a question concerning family history.

15. Do you have a family history of adrenal fatigue?

    ❑ Yes   ❑ No

Childhood history

The use of steroids during your childhood years or prolonged childhood illness may be risk factors for adrenal fatigue.

16. Do you have a history of multiple respiratory infections as a child?

    ❑ Yes   ❑ No

17. Were you ever given steroids as a child?

    ❑ Yes   ❑ No

18. Did you use a steroid inhaler as a child?

    ❑ Yes   ❑ No

    If so, for how many years? _____

19. Did you have any prolonged illness or sickness as a child?

    ❑ Yes   ❑ No

Symptoms

Certain signs and symptoms are associated with adrenal fatigue. This section asks you to report your symptoms.

20. Do you have any of the following symptoms of adrenal fatigue?

Constant weakness and fatigue	❏ Yes	❏ No
Craving salt	❏ Yes	❏ No
Decreased libido	❏ Yes	❏ No
Difficulty sleeping	❏ Yes	❏ No
Getting dizzy when you stand up	❏ Yes	❏ No
Low blood pressure	❏ Yes	❏ No
Low blood sugar	❏ Yes	❏ No
Waking up in the morning feeling exhausted	❏ Yes	❏ No

Dietary history

Consumption of certain foods and beverages increases the risk of developing adrenal fatigue. In this section, you answer questions based on your dietary habits.

21. How many servings of fruits and vegetables do you eat a day? _____

22. Do you consider your diet high in sugar?

    ❏ Yes   ❏ No

23. Do you drink more than two caffeinated beverages a day?

    ❏ Yes   ❏ No

24. Do you drink carbonated beverages?

    ❏ Yes   ❏ No

25. Do you take energy drinks or use energy stimulants?

    ❏ Yes   ❏ No

Work history

Your work environment can be a direct cause of stress and adrenal fatigue. In this section, you answer questions concerning certain aspects of your job.

26. Do you work in any of the following areas?

Medical or health	❏ Yes	❏ No
Sales or retail	❏ Yes	❏ No
Music	❏ Yes	❏ No
Military	❏ Yes	❏ No

27. Do you work more than 8 hours a day?

    ❑ Yes   ❑ No

28. Do you work the night shift?

    ❑ Yes   ❑ No

Sleep history

Adrenal fatigue is associated with poor sleep. This section asks questions concerning your sleep habits.

29. How many hours of sleep do you get a night? (Or if you work a night shift, how many hours do you sleep per day?) _____

30. Have you been diagnosed with sleep apnea?

    ❑ Yes   ❑ No

31. Does your significant other complain about your snoring or kicking in your sleep?

    ❑ Yes   ❑ No

Assessing risk factors and tallying the results

After you fill out the preceding questionnaire, the next step is to evaluate your risk factors and current/potential medical conditions that can cause adrenal fatigue. The following list goes through the various sections of the questionnaire.

✔ **Medical history:** Most adults (we're sorry to say) have at least four chronic illnesses. If you checked off more than two medical conditions listed, you're at increased risk for developing adrenal fatigue. Respiratory conditions (such as asthma, emphysema, and cystic fibrosis) tend to be *recurrent* and require recurrent hospitalizations. They're significant sources of chronic inflammation. Diabetes is known to cause undue stress on many organs, including the eyes, heart, kidneys, nerves, and adrenal glands. Hypothyroidism is a medical condition that's auto-immune in nature, and there's a close connection between thyroid dysfunction and increased adrenal stress.

✔ **Surgical history:** Any type of surgery — even if you've had only one — is a source of acute adrenal stress. The more surgeries you've had in your lifetime, the greater your risk of developing adrenal fatigue later in life. If you needed to have one adrenal gland removed, that places significant stress on the other adrenal gland.

✔ **Medications:** Certain medications, including steroids and pain meds, can increase your risk of developing adrenal fatigue. There's some evidence that statin medications (see Chapter 3) may increase your risk of developing adrenal fatigue.

✔ **Social history:** If you smoke cigarettes, drink more than one alcoholic beverage daily, or use drugs, know that each one of these behaviors is a significant risk factor for developing adrenal fatigue.

✔ **Family history:** Some health professionals have hypothesized that if your family has a history of adrenal fatigue, especially on your mother's side, you're at increased risk of developing adrenal fatigue.

✔ **Childhood history:** Prolonged childhood illness, steroid use as a child, and recurrent childhood infections all increase the risk of developing adrenal fatigue.

✔ **Symptoms:** If you answered three or more of the questions in the symptoms section with a yes, then you most likely have symptomatic adrenal fatigue. (Flip to Chapter 4 for more about adrenal fatigue symptoms.)

✔ **Dietary history:** A diet that's acidic and high in sugar increases your risk of stressing out many organs, especially the adrenal glands. Continued consumption of caffeinated and carbonated beverages is also a no-no for adrenal health. Eating plenty of fruits and vegetables is beneficial.

✔ **Work history:** Certain occupations are at higher risk of causing work-related stress. Working in sales or retail is associated with significant stress. Other high-stress careers include those in the medical and health fields, music, and the military. Even night work can be a stressor.

✔ **Sleep history:** Cortisol secretion is intimately related to sleep, your circadian rhythms, and stress. If you get less than 7 hours of sleep per night, and if the quality of the sleep you do get is poor, you may develop adrenal fatigue. Your lack of sleep also increases your risk of developing weight gain, diabetes, and other chronic illnesses.

Not only is lack of sleep associated with the development of adrenal fatigue and increased cortisol production, but the reverse is also true: In someone with adrenal fatigue, the increase in cortisol production can decrease both sleep quality and sleep quantity.

In addition to seeing how you answered individual sections (Sleep history, Symptoms, and so forth), calculate the total number of answers you marked *yes* to assess your adrenal fatigue risk:

✔ **If your score is greater than 20:** If your total number of yeses is greater than 20, you most likely have adrenal fatigue. You can correct some of the areas where you checked yes — work on them along with the help of your holistic health practitioner and this book.

✔ **If your score is 10 to 20:** You're at high risk of developing adrenal fatigue. Look at the questionnaire again to assess your risk factors and think about how you can reduce or eliminate the risks. That's what a large part of this book is about.

✔ **If your score is less than 10:** You're at mild to moderate risk of developing adrenal fatigue. Identify those areas you marked *yes* and look for the corresponding chapter to find out how you can make positive changes to improve your adrenal health. If you identified work as a source of stress, for example, read Chapter 13 for ways to reduce stress at work. If you marked *yes* to questions on dietary habits, refer to Chapters 9, 12, and 14 through 17 to look for ways to improve your dietary habits and decrease your risk of developing adrenal fatigue.

Don't forget to bring this adrenal fatigue questionnaire with you and discuss the results your healthcare practitioner.

Testing Your Hormones for Adrenal Fatigue

This section focuses on the ways healthcare practitioners test for adrenal fatigue by focusing on hormones produced by the adrenal glands and other parts of the body. Different practitioners have different approaches to evaluating the condition. You need to be aware of the various modes of testing — including blood, urine, and salivary testing — and the advantages of each.

Be sure that you get copies of all your lab work and keep a file for yourself. That way, you have a copy of your medical record and can bring the results with you when you visit your healthcare practitioner. If you have a medical emergency, having all your medical information with you can provide the doctors with all the info they need to give you the best care possible.

Measuring cortisol levels

If your doctor is evaluating your adrenal health, the doc will likely order and evaluate blood and urine tests to measure your cortisol levels. (*Cortisol* has anti-inflammatory properties, helps regulate blood glucose levels, and helps regulate blood pressure. See Chapter 2 for details.)

Just because a blood or urine test comes back normal doesn't mean that adrenal fatigue isn't present. I (coauthor Rich) believe that salivary testing is the way to go when evaluating cortisol levels and other hormone levels as well. Salivary tests provide a more accurate measurement of cortisol deficiency than blood levels do. That doesn't mean that the blood levels are without value, however.

That being said, the first test that health practitioners order is often a morning (AM) cortisol test, which is a blood test. This section describes this test and other ways to measure cortisol.

Understanding morning cortisol

Cortisol is the predominant hormone secreted by the adrenal glands. The morning (AM) cortisol blood test takes place at a lab around 8:00 or 9:00 a.m. — the best time to obtain a blood cortisol level, because your body normally makes (or should make) the highest amount of cortisol in the morning.

In the setting of adrenal fatigue, you'd expect that this test would show a lower than normal cortisol level. In the later stages of adrenal fatigue, you'd expect to find a very low morning cortisol level. A normal range for a blood cortisol level is 5 to 25 micrograms per deciliter (mcg/dL). A level greater than 20 means that your adrenal glands are functioning normally. A level of less than 5 is thought to be a sign of nonfunctioning adrenal glands — the adrenal glands are making little or no cortisol.

If the test comes back with a level between 5 and 20, physicians may find the level hard to interpret — to what degree are the adrenal glands functioning? I (coauthor Rich) think that levels between 5 and 20 may be a sign of adrenal fatigue, but other forms of testing need to be done. AM cortisol isn't a bad test, but it's just a start.

Stimulating the adrenal glands with cosyntropin

When a morning cortisol level is between 5 and 20, doctors may order a cosyntropin stimulation test for more information. *Cosyntropin* is a synthetic copy of the hormone ACTH, which is normally made by the pituitary gland. This hormone stimulates the adrenal glands to make cortisol.

In this test, cosyntropin is given intravenously, and the cortisol levels are measured at 30 minutes and 60 minutes. The cosyntropin should stimulate the adrenal glands enough that the cortisol level doubles. If it doesn't, that may be a sign of absolute adrenal insufficiency.

If you have adrenal fatigue, you may still have a normal cosyntropin stimulation test. The cosyntropin can stimulate the adrenal glands for a short time to give you a normal result. The test provides only a snapshot of adrenal gland functioning; it's too much of a short-term test to provide full value in the diagnosis of adrenal fatigue. Because the test can't completely evaluate for adrenal fatigue, you need further workups. I (coauthor Rich) believe that although this form of testing has some inherent value, salivary testing has more value.

Blood versus salivary testing is a controversial point among many practitioners. Some favor blood testing, which is why we discuss blood testing in this section.

Measuring urinary levels of cortisol

Some healthcare practitioners order urinary cortisol levels. This test is usually done as part of a 24-hour urinary collection (you void into a jug). In most cases, in the setting of adrenal fatigue, the urinary levels of cortisol are lower than one would expect.

A normal urinary level of cortisol is 50 micrograms. Levels less than 10 micrograms are considered suggestive of adrenal fatigue. Unfortunately, like blood tests, urinary tests don't accurately depict the variation of cortisol secretion that occurs over a 24-hour period. This is why salivary testing (see the next section) is so useful.

Testing for salivary cortisol

Blood and urinary tests give you an average of what the adrenal glands are doing over a 24-hour period. Salivary cortisol measurements are better because they give you a sense of the cortisol levels at different times in a 24-hour period.

For the salivary cortisol test, you collect saliva samples at home and send them to a lab for analysis. Your healthcare practitioner will likely recommend a lab where you can get the salivary testing kit. You take saliva samples several times a day, including in the morning, at lunch, at dinner, and before you go to bed. You should also consider collecting a sample when you're experiencing symptoms of adrenal fatigue (see Chapter 4).

Each time you obtain a sample for the salivary cortisol test, you should document how you feel. Your healthcare practitioner's interpretation of many of these levels will be based on how you felt at the time of each sample. The test is very personalized.

You can actually buy a home testing kit on Amazon.com. However, some states have rules about mailing lab tests and medical samples. In California, for example, you have to send in "a written order from a health care professional licensed in California to order laboratory tests."

After collecting samples, you send the saliva to the company that sold you the kit and wait for the results. A normal range for salivary cortisol levels is 20 to 25 nanomoles per liter (nmol/L) in the morning. The salivary cortisol levels decrease throughout the day.

Many labs offer interpretation of the salivary cortisol lab results, but it's imperative that you discuss the results with your healthcare practitioner. Not only are the absolute values of the cortisol levels important, but so is correlating the cortisol levels with how you felt when you collected the samples.

Testing for other adrenal hormones

Besides cortisol, the other adrenal hormones to test for are DHEA, aldosterone, estrogen, pregnenolone, and progesterone (all discussed in Chapter 2). They can be measured in the blood, but I (coauthor Rich) prefer salivary tests because they show how the hormone levels change throughout the day.

For these tests, most healthcare practitioners order a *salivary hormonal profile;* in addition to cortisol, they're ordering levels of DHEA-S (dehydro-epiandrosterone sulfate), estradiol, progesterone, and testosterone. These levels can be tested together.

The interpretation of the hormone testing doesn't just depend on the hormonal levels as measured in the saliva. Hormonal analysis and treatment is much more than simply replacing levels that are low. Your holistic healthcare practitioner will look at your particular hormonal pattern. For example, in many cases of adrenal fatigue, cortisol levels tend to be high and DHEA levels tend to be low.

The levels of the other hormones (estradiol and progesterone) are important as well. Estradiol and progesterone, if needed, have to be prescribed to be in a specific ratio to one another to maintain hormonal balance. Some people may have more of a propensity to convert testosterone to estradiol than others; in these people, for example, testosterone supplementation may not be warranted.

Everyone with adrenal fatigue can have different hormonal patterns and can have different hormonal needs for supplementation. Your healthcare practitioner will review the results of your salivary hormonal analysis in detail. (Refer to Chapter 10 to read about bioidentical hormone supplementation.)

To provide you with some basis for reference, here are average salivary hormonal levels for a typical young man or young woman:

- ✔ **DHEA-S:** A normal DHEA-S range is approximately 7 to 10 nanograms per milliliter (ng/mL) for a man and 3 to 5 ng/mL for a woman.

- ✔ **Estradiol:** A normal estradiol range for a woman is usually around 2 to 2.5 picograms per milliliter (pg/mL). For a man, the normal level is about 0.5 to 1.2 pg/mL.

- ✔ **Testosterone:** A normal level of testosterone is 150 to 200 pg /mL for a man and 25 to 50 pg/mL for a woman.

- ✔ **Progesterone:** A normal range of progesterone is 20 to 50 pg/mL for a man and 70 to 150 pg/mL for a woman.

Testing other important areas

When you're being tested for adrenal fatigue, other testing needs to be done in addition to the hormone testing we discuss in the preceding sections. Specifically, you need to have your thyroid, liver, and kidney function assessed. Here are some tests that do just that:

- ✔ **AM cortisol with an ACTH level:** This blood test can provide information on the status of your pituitary gland. It measures both cortisol and ACTH (adrenocorticotropin hormone) levels. Note that this test differs from the cosyntropin stimulation test we mention earlier.

- ✔ **A TSH with a free T4 (thyroxine) level and free T3 (triiodothyronine) level:** Because the thyroid affects your adrenal glands, your healthcare practitioner should evaluate your thyroid function. The TSH, free T4, and free T3 test helps evaluate the thyroid and pituitary gland.

- ✔ **A serum creatinine level and blood urea nitrogen (BUN) level:** This test evaluates kidney function. Abnormal kidney function can increase the stress and workload on the adrenal glands. Kidney function is often associated with worsening acidosis, which is a direct cause of adrenal stress.

- ✔ **Liver function tests:** These tests help assess liver function. The presence of liver disease can affect the ability of the adrenal glands to produce cortisol.

Evaluating Your Acid-Base Balance

Acidosis (extra acid in the body) can be a potent stimulus and cause of adrenal fatigue. The measure of acidity is pH (see Chapter 2 for details). Because acidosis is a stimulus of inflammation in adrenal fatigue, assessing your body's pH is essential for developing a treatment plan for returning the body's pH to normal. Restoration of a slightly alkaline pH will decrease adrenal gland stress. In this section, we introduce several methods of testing pH.

Measuring acidosis in the blood

Your healthcare provider can order two blood tests to get a sense of how acidic your blood is. The first test is a *serum (blood) bicarbonate level*. The level of bicarbonate (a base) is often measured in the routine blood work that your doctor orders. It's often part of a lab chemistry panel called a *CHEM-7* or a *basic metabolic panel*.

A normal reference range for a serum bicarbonate level in the blood is 23 to 27 milliequivalents per liter (mEq/L). Levels less than 23 suggest that your blood is more acidic than it should be, making it a source of acute adrenal stress.

Other lab chemistries sometimes reveal other conditions that may be causing your blood to be acidic:

✔ **Diabetes:** If your glucose level is really high (a normal level is 70 to 100 milligrams per deciliter or less), an element of diabetes may be causing the acidosis.

✔ **Kidney problems:** If your serum creatinine level is higher than normal, a kidney problem may be contributing to your acidosis. For most people, a serum creatinine less than 1.0 milligram per deciliter means the kidneys are functioning normally.

✔ **Adrenal exhaustion:** If your sodium level is low and your potassium level is high, adrenal exhaustion (see Chapter 4) may be contributing to your acidosis. The range for a normal sodium level in the blood is 135 to 140 mEq/L. The normal potassium range in the blood is 3.5 to 5.0 mEq/L.

The second pH test is a check of the blood's pH level. A normal pH is approximately 7.36. Anything less than that is acidic. I (coauthor Rich) *may* order a pH from blood initially, in addition to other serum chemistries, if multiple reasons suggest that the body is acidic. However, blood pH isn't a test I routinely order.

Looking at urinary pH levels

Of all the types of tests that look for acidosis, I (coauthor Rich) like the urinary pH test the best. It's easy to do, and it measures the body's pH status more accurately than other tests. You can do a urinary pH test either at your healthcare provider's office or at home:

✔ **At the doctor's office:** If you go to the doctor's office, he or she can often do a urinalysis right there. It measures many things, including urine pH, glucose, protein, and blood.

If you go to a lab and get the popular UA (urinary analysis) to include a pH, the urine pH may not accurately reflect your body's chemistry. If your urine sample sits too long, it can become more acidic — and a lab technician may have many urinalyses to process. I consider measuring in real time to be better.

✔ **At home:** You can use many urine pH kits at home. You can urinate in a small cup and dip a pH testing strip in it, or you can void directly on the testing strip. Talk with your holistic healthcare practitioner about which urine pH testing strips are right for you.

Your urinary pH should be approximately 6.5 to 7.0. That's the goal. Expect it to be lower (more acidic) until you begin to change your diet and body chemistry.

At the bare minimum, you want to check your urinary pH first thing in the morning. The urine pH will be the most acidic in the morning and more reflective of your body's true acid-base status. You also can (and should) check it at least once in the afternoon and once in the evening. The food and drink that you consume can alter your urine pH. You want to see how close you are to maintaining your urine pH to 6.5 to 7.0 range, not only in the morning but throughout the day as well.

Checking out the health of the "big three" organs

If your lungs, kidneys, or liver is ill, normalizing your body pH is difficult, no matter what changes you make in your diet or other routines. That's because these organs are essential for eliminating excess acid. Any significant illness that affects the function of these three organs can increase total body acidity (and increase adrenal stress):

- **Lungs:** Your lungs and kidneys work in tandem to help maintain acid-base balance. The lungs eliminate carbon dioxide, and the kidneys eliminate excess acid. Lung conditions that hamper the lungs' ability to get rid of the excess carbon dioxide can cause a *persistent acidosis*. Those conditions include COPD (chronic obstructive pulmonary disease, such as emphysema and chronic bronchitis), chronic asthma, and pneumonia.

- **Kidneys:** Really bad kidney problems such as diabetes and acute kidney failure can also cause acidosis, because the kidneys are unable to eliminate all the acid that has built up in your body.

- **Liver:** Your liver is responsible for regenerating over 80 percent of the bicarbonate in the body. Bicarbonate is a base (the opposite of an acid) whose presence reduces acidity in the body. In advanced liver disease, the liver may not be able to do this function.

The blood work we describe earlier in the chapter can be used to evaluate liver and kidney function. Imaging studies such as a chest X-ray can be done to examine the lungs.

If you're told that you're acidic, ask your healthcare practitioner whether these three organs are healthy. Your healthcare practitioner will likely order blood testing to evaluate your liver and kidney function and discuss what you can do to optimize their functioning. See Chapter 20 for tips.

Investigating Inflammation and Infection

Many conditions can cause and contribute to adrenal fatigue, but inflammation and infection are among the leaders. In this section, you read about ways to test for these conditions. By diagnosing and treating these conditions, you're helping your adrenal glands by decreasing adrenal stress.

The basics: Examining the ESR and C-reactive protein

ESR stands for *erythrocyte sedimentation rate*. It's a blood test, and it's one of the first tests that healthcare practitioners typically order to get a sense whether someone is "inflamed." The normal range for this test is 0 to 20. Most chronic infections and inflammatory syndromes have abnormal sed rates that run in the 80 to 100 range. ***Note:*** This test is nonspecific; it just helps to confirm that there's badness going on without indicating what that badness is.

The test for C-reactive protein (CRP) is often ordered in conjunction with the ESR test to evaluate the presence of an inflammatory or infectious condition. CRP is a protein that reacts to inflammation. The normal range for this test is 1 to 3. In my experience, it's not uncommon in the setting of inflammation or infection to have a level greater than 90.

Testing for rheumatologic and infectious conditions

Beyond the ESR and CRP tests, your healthcare practitioner may order more-specific tests to determine whether inflammation and infection are present. Some of the initial testing that many healthcare providers do includes searching for the rheumatologic conditions (connective tissue diseases) that we discuss in Chapter 7. Here are some typical tests for these conditions:

- ✔ **ANA:** Many docs use the anti-nuclear antibodies (ANA) test to screen for rheumatologic conditions. If the test is positive, the patient needs further evaluation for conditions such as lupus (also known as *systemic lupus erythematosus,* or SLE).
- ✔ **Anti-dsDNA:** This blood test is used to evaluate for lupus.
- ✔ **Rheumatoid factor:** This blood test may be positive in many rheumatologic conditions, including rheumatoid arthritis and lupus.

- ✔ **Anti-RNP:** This is a blood test for mixed connective tissue disease (MCTD), or Sharp's syndrome, in which the person has a little bit of each rheumatologic condition.

- ✔ **Anti-gliadin antibodies or tissue transglutaminase (anti-tTG antibodies):** These blood tests evaluate for the presence of celiac disease.

- ✔ **CPK:** Creatine phosphokinase (CPK for short) is a blood test that's often ordered as part of testing panels. High levels of CPK often indicate some process causing muscle damage of some type.

Here are five tests for infections:

- ✔ **Lyme titer:** This blood test looks for Lyme disease, a chronic infection that can be debilitating. (See Chapter 7 for details on this disease.)

- ✔ **EBV titer (mono spot):** This blood test is for mononucleosis. Viruses can be a root cause of incessant fatigue and weakness. For some people, mono takes months to recover from. I (coauthor Rich) believe that some of this is due to weakened adrenal glands.

- ✔ **HIV (human immunodeficiency virus):** This blood test is good if the patient has certain risk factors for HIV, such as sharing needles and/or unprotected sexual relations with multiple partners.

Looking iridology right in the eye

Your eyes aren't just the windows to your soul; they may also be windows to what's causing an underlying illness. One of the most underused tests in the search for inflammation is *iridology* — examining your iris for patterns, colors, and other characteristics to evaluate your health.

Think of your iris as an illness marker. It's a road map that iridologists use to identify changes in the human body. A good iridology practitioner is able to pinpoint organs that aren't functioning optimally or identify an illness or condition whose symptoms may not yet be evident. I (coauthor Rich) underwent an iridology exam, and I was so surprised at the little things about my health profile that the iridologist found. It picked up even small changes, such as the minor arthritis in my left knee.

I recommend iridology as an additional means of investigation for anyone who has inflammation for which the cause remains elusive. I also recommend it for someone who may be at high risk for developing adrenal fatigue, because iridology can evaluate adrenal function.

This examination probably won't be covered by your health insurance. An average iridology test plus the interpretation of the results can run approximately $100 to $200 per session. In terms of follow-up tests, many practitioners recommend getting a yearly examination. Talk with your healthcare practitioner about whether you need an iridology examination and who he or she would recommend.

✔ **Chronic respiratory infections:** You may need a chest X-ray and sputum culture. With this test, the practitioner looks for specific organisms causing respiratory infections. Such infections need to be treated holistically (looking at all contributing factors) and aggressively.

✔ **Bone imaging:** This includes X-rays and other imaging that may be needed to find *osteomyelitis,* a common type of bone infection. Osteomyelitis is usually due to diabetes.

Testing for environmental toxins

Blood work can be useful in telling you that inflammation is present, and it can be useful in identifying potential causes of that inflammation. But more often than not, more-detailed testing is needed to investigate other causes of inflammation. A significant cause of inflammation is environmental toxins.

Listing environmental toxins

Which toxins are potent stimulators of inflammation? Well, there are many candidates, and they include the following:

✔ Heavy metals, including mercury, arsenic, lead, and cadmium (in particular, mercury is one of the most common causes of heavy metal toxicity and inflammation; see the nearby sidebar for details)

✔ Plastics, such as bisphenol A (BPA), which can affect the integrity of your endocrine system

✔ Toxins and other pollutants in the food you eat

✔ Cleaning supplies, including laundry detergent

✔ Food allergens and sensitivities that can be evaluated through blood testing (see Chapter 8)

Environmental toxins affect people all the time. Understand that chronic inflammation and illness from toxin exposure is a result of cumulative exposure over months or years. Environmental toxins have been linked to many chronic illnesses, such as rheumatoid arthritis, lupus, diabetes, and cancer.

Toxins can also cause weight gain. BPA is a toxin in plastic that's referred to as a *hormonal manipulator.* It can simulate the actions of estrogen, with weight gain being a significant side effect. Note that although weight gain is mostly affected by diet and exercise (or lack thereof), the science of obesity has demonstrated that toxins and fungal overgrowth (see Chapter 8) also play a role in weight gain. Fat cells are treasure chests of inflammatory proteins. For many people, obesity contributes to the development of adrenal fatigue through its stimulation of the inflammatory process.

Undergoing hair testing for toxins

Just measuring blood levels of a particular toxin, especially heavy metals, won't give you any information about the degree of toxicity in the tissues. Some healthcare practitioners do a *chelation test.* This test involves giving you a substance like EDTA (ethylenediaminetetraacetic acid), which removes some of the metals from your tissues and puts them in the bloodstream. The next step is a 24-hour urine collection to quantitate the metals excreted.

The urine collection for a chelation test is very complicated. In fact, it's so cumbersome that patients often don't do it correctly, so as a kidney doctor, I try to limit the number of 24-hour urine collections done.

Because toxins go deep into the tissues, performing a hair analysis is one of the best ways to get a sense of tissue toxicity. A hair analysis is easy to do (it can be done at home) and is noninvasive. The only requirements are that you have hair and don't live in the state of New York, because this testing isn't allowed there!

Mentioning mercury

I (coauthor Rich) believe that all healthcare practitioners should test for levels of mercury and other heavy metals (manganese, aluminum, cadmium, beryllium, and arsenic). Mercury toxicity has been linked to many chronic diseases, including inflammatory arthritis, cancer, neuropathy, heart disease, and stroke. Other consequences of heavy metal toxicity include liver and kidney disease.

Mercury causes its toxic effects by interfering with the activities of the cell. It enters a cell, interferes with chemical reactions, and depletes the body of trace minerals such as zinc. It also causes a rapid depletion of potent cellular antioxidants, including glutathione.

With regard to heavy metals, you can take all the antioxidants that you want, but unless you do something to eliminate the heavy metal load, the anti-inflammatories and antioxidants won't be very effective. Chelation is an effective way of eliminating heavy metals from the body. For information concerning chelation, visit the National Capital Poison Center website at www.poison.org/current/chelationtherapy.htm.

Note: Be aware that many older dental fillings contain mercury. Fortunately, most dentists no longer use mercury amalgam. Just the same, it's a smart idea to ask your dentist not to use this toxin in your fillings.

A hair analysis can measure metals, minerals, and electrolytes. Just from the hair sample, a lab quantifies the amounts of each toxin or nutrient in the body:

- ✔ **Metals:** Mercury, lead, arsenic, and cadmium
- ✔ **Minerals:** Zinc, magnesium, calcium, selenium, and manganese
- ✔ **Electrolytes:** Potassium and phosphorous

Together, the levels of all these substances provide a profile that can tell you and your healthcare practitioner many things. It's not by accident that "heavy metal poisoning" is in the modern vocabulary.

Don't wash your hair before collecting the hair sample, because washing may affect the results. (Here's the kicker: Some labs wash the hair sample that you send to them, which may affect the reliability of the test.) Cut your hair as close to the scalp as possible for the best possible result. If you're bald, you can still have this test done using hair from other areas (you get the gist).

After the test is done, the testing center should offer you the opportunity to have a review session with an individual who specializes in the interpretation of the hair analysis. In an ideal world, your healthcare practitioner would want to speak with this specialist to determine how best to personalize your treatment regimen. However, many health practitioners are reluctant to even order the test, let alone speak with such a specialist. You need to be an advocate for your own health and treatment. In terms of price, many of these tests can range from $100 to $300.

What's in your water?

Have you ever looked at the results of a water test? There's a lot of stuff in tap water that shouldn't be there. When you review the results of such a test, you may read that the toxins are "within acceptable levels." That should be your first clue that something is wrong. Metals, toxins, pesticide/herbicide residues, remnants of medications (people will flush anything down the toilet), and just about everything else is likely to make your water toxic.

You can call your township or county to get the results of its most recent water testing. You may not like what you hear. Given that your body is 70 percent water and that water bathes the cells in your body, you should know what's in your water and expect a reasonable level of purity.

In Chapter 11, you read about alkaline water. Drinking alkaline water is a good way to modify your water intake, especially if you don't use tap water, as some online sources recommend. At the very least, you need a filter for your tap water. Anything is better than nothing.

Putting It All Together and Making the Diagnosis

In this chapter, you read about testing for adrenal fatigue. The exhaustive adrenal fatigue questionnaire is the first part of the journey, because it not only looks for signs and symptoms of adrenal fatigue but also identifies risk factors and dietary and lifestyle habits that increase the risk of developing adrenal fatigue.

The key test that confirms the diagnosis of adrenal fatigue is the salivary hormone test, particularly the salivary cortisol test. If this test is positive, the next step is to identify the risk factors in your life that caused you to develop adrenal fatigue. With this information, you and your healthcare practitioner can develop a personalized treatment plan not only to help you overcome adrenal fatigue but also to reduce adrenal stress and develop strategies to prevent adrenal fatigue from occurring in the future.

Part II
Getting a Handle on Potential Trigger Factors

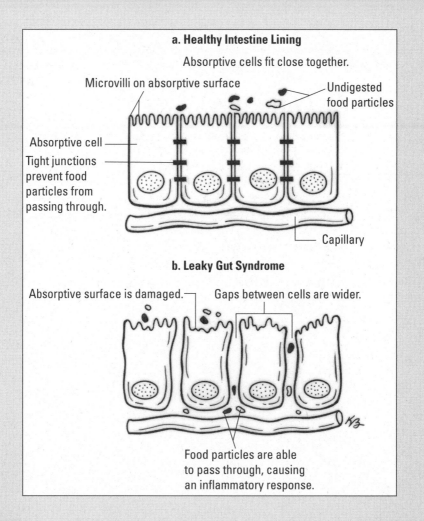

a. Healthy Intestine Lining

Absorptive cells fit close together.

Microvilli on absorptive surface

Undigested food particles

Absorptive cell

Tight junctions prevent food particles from passing through.

Capillary

b. Leaky Gut Syndrome

Absorptive surface is damaged.

Gaps between cells are wider.

Food particles are able to pass through, causing an inflammatory response.

Discover the connection between adrenal fatigue and intestinal health in an article at www.dummies.com/extras/adrenalfatigue.

In this part...

- ✔ Understand how stress and lack of sleep contribute to adrenal fatigue and discover what you can do to combat them. Over time, trying to maintain a crazy (and destructive) pace with too much stress and too little sleep can cause both you and your adrenal glands to become completely exhausted.

- ✔ See how chronic inflammation and acidosis are strongly associated with the development of adrenal fatigue, and get tips on how to combat their causes.

- ✔ Investigate the major role of the intestine in immune system regulation, and find out about key nutrients that are necessary for boosting adrenal health.

Chapter 6

The Effects of Stressing Out and Sleeping Less

In This Chapter

▶ Seeing how stress affects your adrenal glands

▶ Sleeping better to give your adrenal glands a break

*I*n this modern, fast-paced world, two of the biggest contributing factors to adrenal fatigue are chronic stress and lack of sleep. People work too hard and relax too little. They don't sleep as long as they would like to or should. Over time, trying to maintain this crazy (and destructive) pace can cause both you and your adrenal glands to become fatigued and even completely exhausted.

In this chapter, you read about the importance of reducing stress and sleeping better — if you don't make some lifestyle changes, you can potentially exhaust your adrenal glands completely. You also find some tips on lowering stress and getting a good night's sleep.

Connecting Stress to Adrenal Fatigue

Stress is a significant contributor to adrenal fatigue. What exactly is stress? It's difficult to quantify, but you know when you're under stress. One commonly used definition of *stress* is how you physically and/or emotionally respond to stimuli. Stressors can be external (your environment) or internal (your thoughts or emotions). You're usually reacting to multiple stressors at any given time.

Constant stress throws your body out of balance and affects the functioning of many glands, especially the adrenal glands. In this section, we note some typical stressors, symptoms of chronic stress, and methods for reducing stress.

Examining common stressors

If stress is so bad, then why does your body have the ability to be stressed at all? Well, *acute* stress can be beneficial and actually life-saving. The goal of the fight-or-flight reaction is self-preservation.

Imagine for a second that you're living in prehistoric times being chased by a wild boar. Your fight-or-flight reaction kicks in because you're running for your life. This stress reaction ends when you climb a tree to escape or figure out a way to trap and kill the boar. This is an example of a normal or *physiologic stress,* and your reaction helps keep you alive.

In modern times, you may have an acute stress response when fleeing from an attacker or trying to avoid a car crash. In those situations, your pupils dilate, your heart rate increases, and your endurance and reflex capabilities are maximized so you can run farther and faster away from your attacker or turn to avoid the crash. Here, the acute stress saves your life.

Compare these scenarios to the constant sources of stress in modern daily life. You face personal, family, and work stressors, and even your cellphone and other electronic devices can be sources of electromagnetic stress.

You can probably relate in some way to the following scenario: You jump out of bed at the sound of a buzzer, still exhausted because you got only 6 hours of sleep. You quickly dress, rush to get out the door, and figure you'll grab breakfast on the way. Maybe you say goodbye to your significant other and kids, or maybe you fly out the door and miss them entirely. You go to your local coffee spot and grab a large morning coffee (the Super Jolt) as well as a doughnut, bear claw, or other sugary substance.

You drive to work, fervently looking at the time, hoping to make that next light so you won't be late. You miss the light and begin to curse at the person in front of you traveling 20 mph in a 55 mph zone. You may add a couple of angry honks for good measure. You barely make it to work on time and wait with a mob of people for the elevators. Although you work on only the third floor, you avoid the exercise of running up the stairs (if you have adrenal fatigue, you're simply too tired). You mutter under your breath because the elevator is running slow.

You spend the rest of your day stressing out over deadlines; you work through lunch and through your breaks. You deal with various memos and bosses who don't have a clue about what the heck you do all day. You may even work late and grab something from the drive-through at your local burger joint on the way home. You drive home, exhausted, and still get little sleep. The next day begins like the previous one.

For most people, this is what a typical day consists of: chronic stress, poor sleep, inadequate nutrition, little or no exercise, and increased inflammation. Their adrenal glands never get a chance to rest and recuperate.

Surveying the symptoms of chronic stress

To deal with a constant barrage of stress, your adrenal glands are producing mega amounts of hormones, especially cortisol. Your adrenal glands eventually become fatigued; they simply can't keep up with the demand that the continued stress has placed on them. (In Chapter 2, you read about the detrimental effects to the body that persistently high levels of cortisol can cause over time.)

People also make unhealthy choices as they go throughout their day, increasing their stress. Poor nutrition (lack of breakfast and/or lunch), lack of exercise (taking the elevator instead of the stairs), not taking any breaks during the day (no chance to meditate, walk during lunch, and/or take any time for themselves) — these poor choices only exhaust the adrenal gland reserves even further. They deplete already depleted adrenal glands.

Many people are so entrenched in the comings and goings of their daily lives that they don't recognize symptoms of chronic stress, which may be emotional, mental, or physical:

- ✔ **Emotional:** Emotional symptoms may include anger, depression, or a combination of the two. You may be unable to relax, or you may find yourself tense all the time, ready to jump down someone's throat at the slightest irritation. You may be emotionally fatigued all the time but unable to sleep.

- ✔ **Mental:** Confusion or difficulty concentrating is an often unrecognized symptom of stress. Having problems with short-term memory, feeling stuck, and feeling spacey can also result from chronic stress. You read about brain fog as a symptom of stress in Chapter 4.

- ✔ **Physical:** Physical symptoms include chest pressure and/or pain, palpitations (heart pounding), sweating, nausea, and insomnia.

Anxiety or panic attacks can manifest in a variety of ways, including chest pain and palpitations. Don't ignore these symptoms and simply attribute them to stress or anxiety. If you're experiencing any of these symptoms, you need to be evaluated by a health professional immediately. A lot of medical conditions can cause chest pain and palpitations, angina being the first that comes to mind.

In and out: Breathing to reduce stress

One great way to reduce stress, no matter where you are, is to focus on your breathing. Breathing deeply can inhibit the body's sympathetic tone (the fight-or-flight reaction), decreasing the work of the adrenal glands. It's also a great way to help lower blood pressure, detoxify your body, and calm your thoughts.

How do you breathe effectively? Ideally, you should sit on the floor in a relaxed position, though you can do this exercise standing in an elevator, sitting at your desk, or at a playground watching your kids. Here's what to do:

1. **Take in a deep breath for a count of four.** When you inhale, breathe in through your mouth. Keep your mouth open and breathe with your diaphragm. You'll know you're breathing with your diaphragm when you take in a deep breath and you see your stomach get bigger.

2. **Hold that breath for another count of four.**

3. **Release that breath slowly for another count of four.** Exhale slowly, again through an open mouth.

Repeat this exercise a few times. After about the fourth or fifth deep breath, you should feel the stress leave your body.

The key is to incorporate this breathing into your daily routine until it becomes automatic. Begin by taking a few minutes in the morning or a few minutes during your workday at lunch. Use this breathing technique a few times throughout the day. You should also train yourself to use this technique before knowingly heading into any stressful situation. This exercise takes practice. The more that you do it, the more it will feel like second nature to you.

Reducing stress in your daily life

Here are some general ways to try to reduce stress in your daily life (see Chapter 13 for work-specific tips). These tips don't take a lot of time — we promise!

✔ **Get to the root of the problem.** Why are you so stressed out? Is it work? Is it family? Talk to someone — a trusted friend, a family member, and/or a therapist. Don't shoulder the burden alone. Find out what's causing the stress and how best to deal with it.

If you're able to get some distance from the stressor, that can be immensely helpful. Depending on the nature of the stressor, however, that may not be practical.

✔ **Learn how to say no.** One of the hardest things to understand is that there are only 24 hours in a day. Learning when to say no can be a great way to avoid burnout. The first step is knowing your limits. Understanding when you're maxed out and can't add any more to your plate can help you say no when you're asked to tackle yet another project.

✔ **Enjoy daily exercise.** There's no greater way to relieve stress than with a daily dose of exercise. The exercise that you engage in should help you relieve stress, and it may be enjoyable, too.

What type of exercise should you engage in? Well, you know yourself better than anyone. For some, a solitary bike ride is more than enough to get some exercise and some quality "me time" in the process. For others, a basketball game can do the trick. You know what you need to do. The key is to be sure that you do it.

Check with your healthcare provider before beginning any exercise program; if you have adrenal fatigue or adrenal exhaustion, you may need to modify your exercise plan, or you may need adrenal support. Please refer to Chapter 12 for tips on beginning an exercise program in the setting of adrenal fatigue.

✔ **Take time to breathe deeply.** For tips, check out the nearby sidebar "In and out: Breathing to reduce stress."

✔ **Sleep better.** We cover this in detail in the next section.

✔ **Get some sun daily.** Not only does going outside give you a much-needed break, but it also gives you some sunlight, which allows your body to replenish its vitamin D. Vitamin D levels can help restore your immune system and help your body cope with daily stresses.

✔ **Stay hydrated.** Your body is more than 60 percent water. Staying hydrated is important for keeping cells and tissues healthy, reducing inflammation. Choose filtered and purified water — you don't need to add more toxins to an already stressed-out body. Check out Chapter 11 to read about alkaline water as a suitable choice for your water consumption.

✔ **Avoid relying on the morning coffee.** The caffeine from your morning cup of coffee can be one heck of a jolt to your adrenal glands. Most people don't stop at just one cup. In addition, caffeine can raise blood pressure, make you jittery, and cause dehydration.

✔ **Eliminate the sugar rush.** Not only is sugar a cause of total body inflammation, but it's also a significant stressor on your adrenal glands. Imagine the major stress on the adrenal glands when they're hit with a double dose of both caffeine and sugar.

Sugar substitutes aren't a good substitute for sugar. Aspartame, for example, is associated with weight gain and may increase the risk of developing diabetes. One of the best sources of a natural sweetener that we recommend is stevia.

✔ **Don't smoke.** Cigarettes contain many toxins — including cadmium, mercury, and arsenic — that are just bad for the body. Nicotine increases adrenal stress and can raise blood pressure. Smoking increases total body inflammation as well as atherosclerosis (hardening of the blood vessels) exponentially.

✔ **Ward off electromagnetic radiation.** People are exposed to a lot of electromagnetic radiation, which is a potent source of stress, on a daily basis. This radiation can be a source of constant fatigue, malaise, recurrent infections, and brain fog. Your cellphone, your microwave, the power lines outside your house, and multiple televisions and computers all can be sources of electromagnetic stress.

In addition to being aware of your environment and reducing your exposure to electromagnetic fields, one potential solution is wearing a personal diode. Think of the diode as a filter that protects the body from the effects of radiation. You can wear radiation protection diodes or simply place them in your pocket.

Taking your shoes off

An article from the *Journal of Environmental and Public Health* in 2012 discussed an easy way to de-stress your body and restore balance: Simply take your shoes off. The idea goes like this: The Earth's surface is an enormous source of electrons. Connection with the physical earth on a daily basis is essential for keeping the body healthy. The problem is that many people wear sneakers or insulated footwear for long periods of time, preventing them from being connected to the earth.

Think of your body as a large electrical system. Your cells are normally in an oxidized state or a reduced or natural state. The longer cells are in an oxidized state, the more damage to the cells. Long-term exposure to electromagnetic radiation can exert significant oxidative damage and oxidative stress to your cells. Oxidized cells are more prone to form free radicals, which can further damage cells and tissues. Oxidation is a potent stimulator of total body inflammation.

Some people suggest that one way to normalize your body's electrical system is "earthing." Simply by taking your shoes off and walking barefoot, you're connecting with the earth and grounding yourself. Electrons are transferred from the earth to your body, helping your cells maintain their natural state and minimizing oxidative damage. This increases the health of the blood and reduces total body inflammation.

On a daily basis, simply take your shoes off and walk around outside for a few minutes. Doing this at home, where you're familiar with your surroundings, is probably best. That being said, there's nothing like walking barefoot at the beach!

Linking Sleeplessness to Adrenal Fatigue

During sleep, your body repairs itself and regenerates. Lack of sleep over a period of time weakens your immune system and can affect thinking, mood, and judgment. Long-term sleep deprivation is a risk factor for high blood pressure, coronary artery disease, diabetes, and many chronic illnesses. Lack of sleep has even been shown to cause weight gain.

Sleep deprivation also impairs the functioning of many organs in the body, especially the adrenal glands. One of the best treatments for adrenal fatigue is getting a good night's sleep. In this section, we talk about issues with sleep quantity and quality, and we list ways to improve the sleep you get.

Probing sleep problems

Many people find themselves trying to cram more and more into a 24-hour day. In fact, the average time for sleep at night has decreased by almost 2 hours in the past two decades. The average person gets approximately 6 hours of sleep a night.

Dealing with the night shift

Although most people work during the day, much of the population works during the night and sleeps during the day. These people can include healthcare workers, taxi drivers, truck drivers, data entry workers, casino workers, factory workers, cooks, and bakers, to name a few. There are also many people who work rotating shifts. Switching between day and night shifts can be even more of a challenge in obtaining the rest that you need.

Sleeping during the day can be very difficult, and the demands of the family often limit how much sleep night-shift workers get. Even if they're able to sleep 7 to 8 hours during the day, the quality of sleep may be poor. Many workers actually develop something called *shift work sleep disorder* (SWSD); they have difficulty regulating their sleep rhythms with their work schedule. An article from the *Journal of Clinical Psychiatry* in 2012 mentioned that shift work

sleep disorder increases the risk of developing other health problems, including cancer and heart disease.

Here are some tips for improving your sleep if you work nights:

- ✔ One of the keys to treatment is trying to get into as regular a sleep pattern as you can. Try to keep the same sleep schedule every day.

- ✔ Achieve a minimum of 6 hours of sleep each day if possible.

- ✔ When sleeping during the day, try to mimic nighttime by covering the windows to reduce the amount of light coming into the room.

- ✔ Consider using supplements, such as valerian root and melatonin, that can help you get a "good day's sleep." Refer to Chapter 11 for information on these supplements.

Maybe you're one of the lucky few who are able to get 7 or 8 hours a night, but you awaken and feel as if you haven't slept at all. In fact, you feel like you could sleep another 8 hours. The following things may affect your ability to get a good night's sleep:

✓ **Staying up late to engage in activities:** Many people like to stay up to enjoy some personal time after the rest of the family has turned in. You can get caught up watching TV, surfing the Internet, text messaging, and reading, among other activities. Keep in mind how long you spend on these activities and whether they're affecting the amount of time you spend sleeping.

✓ **Stress:** Stress can be a major reason you can't sleep at night. We cover stress in depth earlier in this chapter.

✓ **Pain and chronic illness:** Many causes of adrenal fatigue are also associated with pain and chronic illness. They include fibromyalgia, chronic pain syndrome, and many rheumatologic conditions, such as systemic lupus erythematosus (SLE) and rheumatoid arthritis (RA).

✓ **Food and nutrient deficiencies:** The issue of food and sleep involves much more than not eating a few hours before you go to bed. Certain foods can be a cause of food sensitivities, which promote inflammation and stress.

Nutrient deficiencies can also impair your sleep:

• Low magnesium levels can be associated with your inability to get a good night's sleep. Low magnesium levels often aren't associated with symptoms; however, severe magnesium deficiency can be associated with symptoms such as muscle weakness and cramping.

• Iron deficiency can be associated with restless legs syndrome. People with this condition report feeling numbness and tingling; they feel as if their legs "want to go dancing" while the rest of them wants to go to sleep.

✓ **Hormonal imbalances:** Imbalances can affect the quality and quantity of sleep. Low levels of estrogen, in particular, are closely related to insomnia.

✓ **Sleep apnea:** Sleep apnea is one of the most common causes of poor sleep. Recognizing the symptoms and treating this condition is paramount in getting a good night's sleep. Refer to the sidebar "Diagnosing and treating sleep apnea" for details.

Poor sleep quantity and quality can increase adrenal stress and cortisol secretion, which can contribute to weight gain. Insufficient sleep is also associated with increased inflammation, which can further stress the adrenal glands. A journal article from the *Annals of the New York Academy of Sciences* in 2006 mentioned that the reverse is also true: If your adrenal glands are producing high amounts of cortisol, the high cortisol levels will affect your ability to get a good night's sleep. This means that an inability to get a good night's sleep is due to a multitude of factors, including your level of adrenal fatigue. A holistic view of health is necessary because poor sleep can be one among many issues that need to be evaluated.

Diagnosing and treating sleep apnea

Have you ever been told that you're a loud snorer? Maybe your significant other noticed you had periods during the night where you seemed to stop breathing for a second or two. Or maybe you sleep for 8 hours, but you wake up feeling exhausted anyway. Maybe every morning when you wake, you have headaches (due to oxygen deprivation). Or perhaps you fall asleep in the middle of the day. If any of these symptoms pertain to you, you may have sleep apnea. Be aware that although snoring is a common symptom of sleep apnea, not everyone with sleep apnea snores loudly.

Sleep apnea is one of the most under-recognized causes of poor sleep quality. It's also linked to high blood pressure that's difficult to get under control, kidney disease, and, believe it or not, adrenal stress. People with sleep apnea essentially aren't getting the oxygen they need at night. They're not only sleep-deprived but also oxygen-deprived.

Here's how I (coauthor Rich) explain this condition to patients: Picture someone partially strangling you every time you go to sleep. Deprived of oxygen, your body goes into a fight-or-flight reaction. Your heart, responding to the oxygen deprivation, works vigorously to pump blood (red blood cells carry oxygen to your body cells). Your lungs work harder as well. Your adrenal glands are working overtime when you sleep, secreting high levels of the hormones epinephrine, aldosterone, and cortisol. To varying degrees, this happens each and every night you go to sleep if you have sleep apnea. You can see how sleep apnea can lead to adrenal fatigue. Many people with sleep apnea go undiagnosed for years.

If your healthcare provider suspects you have sleep apnea, he or she may order a sleep study, or *polysomnography*. This type of testing is performed on an outpatient basis, usually at a sleep center. The pattern of your sleeping is observed to see whether sleep apnea is present.

Sleep apnea is closely linked to obesity, so one of the main treatments for sleep apnea is weight loss. A more immediate treatment is continuous positive airway pressure (CPAP), which involves wearing a face mask that provides you with oxygen while you sleep. For many, the mask can be difficult to tolerate. Refraining from alcohol is also important, because alcohol can worsen sleep apnea symptoms. The key is not to ignore symptoms of sleep apnea, because it can be a major source of undiagnosed fatigue.

Low testosterone can contribute to malaise and fatigue, especially in older men. Some evidence demonstrates that sleep apnea can lower testosterone levels. Correcting sleep apnea may help normalize testosterone levels so that replacement isn't even necessary.

Sleeping longer and better

To sleep longer and better, first be aware of things you can control that may affect your sleep. To improve the quality and quantity of your sleep, try the following tips:

- **Meditate and exercise daily.** They're great ways to reduce stress and can increase your chances of getting a good night's sleep (see the earlier section "Reducing stress in your daily life" for details).

- **Address food sensitivities and nutrient deficiencies.** When you begin to correct nutrient deficiencies and avoid foods that are making you feel bad, your quality of life and your quality of sleep improve. (Please see Chapter 8 for more information on nutrition.)

    - **Magnesium:** Supplementing with magnesium and/or increasing the amount of green vegetables in your diet (which are great sources of magnesium) can improve your sleep.

    - **Iron:** You may need to begin supplementing with iron. Examples of common prescription medications include ferrous sulfate and ferrous gluconate. Talk with your healthcare practitioner about the best iron preparation for you.

        Adding vitamin C to any iron preparation can enhance its absorption. Also be aware that any iron supplement should be taken separately from other medications and supplements because it may affect their absorption.

    In Chapter 11, you read about the various supplements and remedies that you can take to help you sleep better.

- **Avoid eating anything at least 3 to 4 hours before going to bed.** Eating just before you go to bed is a really big no-no. After you eat, your body is busy trying to digest the food; it's not ready to relax and go to sleep. If you lie down soon after eating, you also increase the risk of heartburn that can certainly keep you up at night.

    By the same token, avoid drinking right before going to bed. You may find yourself having to get up more than a few times during the night to use the bathroom.

- **Avoid caffeine:** Make a point to avoid caffeinated beverages because the caffeine, being a stimulant, will make it harder to go to sleep.

- **Relieve inflammation and pain.** Try the techniques in Chapter 11.

- **Pick a quitting time.** In terms of late-night activities, pick a time where you stop the activity and go to bed. This goes for office work, school work, reading, and so on. Getting a good night's sleep will make you more productive the next day.

- **Wear earplugs.** Do you awaken at the slightest noise and then have trouble getting back to sleep? Well, a good set of earplugs may be just what the doctor ordered.

Chapter 7

The Contributions of Inflammation and Acidosis to Adrenal Fatigue

---

---

*T*wo big contributors to the development of adrenal fatigue are inflammation and *acidosis* (acidic blood). In this chapter, we explain how these two conditions can lead to adrenal fatigue and list their common causes. These conditions often occur together because changes in the body's pH balance can promote inflammation.

Clarifying the Role of Inflammation in Adrenal Fatigue

Inflammation is a major cause of many chronic illnesses, including heart disease and cancer. Chronic inflammation is also strongly associated with the development of adrenal fatigue. What exactly is inflammation? This section compares normal inflammation to chronic inflammation, which can lead to adrenal fatigue.

Understanding a normal inflammatory response

Your body's ability to generate an inflammatory response to an acute illness or injury is beneficial to your health. If you get a sore throat, for example, the acute illness stimulates your body's immune system to fight off the infection. If you experience an injury, such as an ankle sprain, your body goes into repair mode. The inflammatory response, which can cause pain and swelling of the ankle, is designed to help the ankle get better. Healthy cells replace the injured cells.

The damage that occurs in the cells as a result of an acute trauma or acute illness causes something called *oxidative stress.* Oxidative stress causes the formation of *free radicals,* which are highly toxic unstable molecules that damage cells. They're a potent stimulus of the body's inflammatory response. The inflammatory response is necessary to deal with the acute injury or illness, eliminate the toxic free radicals that have formed as a result of the injury, and begin the healing process. After a few days, as your body begins to recover from the illness or injury, the body's inflammatory response decreases.

Experiencing a continued inflammatory response

What if your body's inflammatory response never turns off after an illness or injury? Oxidative stress to the cells continues, and more free radicals form, which stimulates the inflammatory response even more. Proteins that stimulate the inflammatory response are commonly referred to as *cytokines.* One class of these proteins is the *interleukins;* they're significant contributors to the sustained inflammation of many chronic illnesses, including cancer and arthritis. This continued inflammatory response can have dire health consequences and is felt to be a significant cause of and contributor to cancer, heart disease, vascular disease, kidney disease, and adrenal fatigue.

With adrenal fatigue in particular, sustained inflammation causes the adrenal glands to secrete more cortisol. Day after day, the adrenal glands are unable to meet the demands that chronic inflammation and chronic stress have on them. The adrenal glands become fatigued and, over time, exhausted.

Poor nutrition, stress, poor sleep, hormonal imbalances, an unhealthy intestinal tract, chronic illnesses (like those in the next section), and acid-base imbalances (like those we describe later in this chapter) are all potent stimulators of the inflammatory response.

Unless chronic inflammation is recognized and treated, the effects can be bad; they can include heart attack and stroke. I (coauthor Rich) believe that everyone has some degree of inflammation because of his or her environment and lifestyle. I think the key to recognizing whether inflammation is present is to see a healthcare practitioner who is holistically minded. See Chapter 9 for information on finding a good practitioner.

Considering Causes of Chronic Inflammation

Several causes of chronic inflammation are strongly associated with the development of adrenal fatigue. They include rheumatologic conditions, potent chronic inflammatory conditions, fibromyalgia, rheumatoid arthritis, and autoimmune disorders like lupus, as well as intestine-related conditions such as celiac disease (which we describe in Chapter 8), endocrine disorders such as thyroid dysfunction, and chronic infections such as Lyme disease. If you have one of these conditions, you're more likely to develop adrenal fatigue. In reality, many people have more than one condition at the time they're diagnosed with adrenal fatigue.

Fighting fibromyalgia syndrome

Fibromyalgia syndrome (FMS) is a medical condition that's really a constellation of symptoms strongly characterized by muscle pain, fatigue, and an inability to get a decent night's sleep. The symptoms of FMS are definitely life-altering and can be debilitating, but treatment is available. In this section, you read about the symptoms and treatment of FMS, and you find information on the potential link between FMS and the adrenal glands.

Although the cause of FMS is unknown, it may be viral or infectious in origin. One study from the medical journal *Clinical and Experimental Rheumatology* in 2011 noted that people who'd been diagnosed with Lyme disease, hepatitis C or B, HIV, or parvovirus had a higher incidence of pain and FMS-type symptoms.

Symptoms

If you've been diagnosed with FMS or strongly suspect that you have it, you may have experienced one or more of the following symptoms for at least 3 months:

- **Diffuse pain, characterized by the presence of multiple tender points throughout the body:** The classic definition of FMS consists of the presence at least 11 out of 18 possible tender points. The tender points are easily detected by applying firm pressure to specific areas of the body.

- **Sleep that isn't restorative:** You can sleep for 10 hours, awaken, and feel as if you haven't slept at all. Often people affected with FMS have trouble falling asleep and suffer from insomnia.

- **Chronic fatigue and exhaustion:** This goes hand in hand with the preceding point concerning sleep; however, any type of strenuous activity can leave someone with FMS completely debilitated, often needing to lie in bed for hours or days.

✔ **Joint pain and headaches:** Joint pain, morning stiffness, and headaches often occur with this syndrome.

✔ **Mental symptoms:** Other symptoms can include difficulties with thinking, trouble concentrating, memory problems, and depression.

In many cases, the symptoms of fibromyalgia overlap with the symptoms of chronic fatigue syndrome (CFS). The two are often grouped together as one syndrome complex. Recognizable symptoms of CFS include extreme fatigue following exercise, difficulty sleeping, recurrent sore throats, headaches, an inability to concentrate, and problems with memory. For a diagnosis of CFS, the symptoms need to persist for at least 6 months.

FMS can occur on its own, or it can occur with conditions such as rheumatoid arthritis and lupus, both of which we discuss later in this chapter.

Sometimes severe psychological or physical stress or trauma can precipitate the onset of acute FMS symptoms. If you have FMS, think back to when you first began to experience the symptoms. Did a significant, perhaps life-changing event occur first? Did you have an acute illness? Did the symptoms start after you received a vaccination? Were you involved in a motor vehicle accident or other significant trauma? Did a family member or significant other pass away?

Treatment

Treating FMS is multifaceted; it involves improving energy, improving nutrition, supplementing when needed, and reducing inflammation:

✔ **Increasing energy:** From a cellular perspective, FMS is energy-sapping. The goal of treatment is to increase the energy to the cell. The following supplements can help in this regard:

  • Ubiquinone (coenzyme Q_{10})

  • D-ribose

  • Magnesium (taken as magnesium malate, the combination of magnesium and malic acid can be a great energy booster to the cell)

You can find these supplements in Chapter 11; we recommend referring to that chapter after you finish reading this section.

  • **Handling hormonal imbalances:** Testing for and correcting hormonal imbalances is paramount in the treatment of FMS. (Correcting hormonal imbalances is also key in the treatment of adrenal fatigue; see Chapter 10 for details.)

  • **Reducing inflammation:** To reduce inflammation, try to normalize your intestine. Looking for and treating fungal overgrowth and promoting healthy intestinal flora is important in the treatment of FMS. (As you read in Chapter 8, normalizing bowel flora is important in treating adrenal fatigue as well). The use of systemic anti-inflammatories and antioxidants can also be very beneficial.

- **Improving nutrition:** Eradicate pro-inflammatory foods, instead choosing foods that are anti-inflammatory and alkaline in nature. Refer to Chapter 8 for information on dietary changes that reduce inflammation.

- **Embracing exercise:** Having FMS doesn't mean you can't exercise. It just means that you need to exercise *the right way.* Please refer to Chapter 12 for information on exercise.

- **Getting some sleep:** If you have FMS, it's so important that you do everything you can to get a good night's sleep. Increasing your magnesium intake, using melatonin, and using herbs such as valerian root may help. The use of prescribed sleep aids is encouraged, too. See Chapter 11 to read about sleep remedies.

A possible connection between FMS and the adrenal glands

Ongoing research is looking at a possible connection between FMS and the adrenal glands. In someone with FMS, the level of activity of the adrenal glands is reduced. A malfunctioning of the adrenal gland receptors is a potential problem.

One study from the journal *Psychoneuroendocrinology* in 2012 evaluated people suffering from FMS-related pain and measured the associated level of cortisol secretion from the adrenal glands. The researchers noted that patients with FMS showed decreased cortisol secretion. The investigators hypothesized that FMS involves a problem with the steroid (cortisol) receptor in the adrenal gland itself. Another study from the journal *Psychosomatic Medicine* in 2008 suggests that adrenal gland activity may be decreased in someone with FMS, as researchers found a decrease in the total cortisol released from the adrenal glands.

Further studies are needed, but research suggests that adrenal gland activity is lessened in patients with FMS. But how much is cause, and how much is effect? How much does FMS or chronic inflammation affect the activity of the adrenal glands over time? Conversely, does a primary issue with the adrenal glands cause an exaggerated response to pain and susceptibility to viral illnesses that predispose certain individuals to develop FMS? For me (coauthor Rich) as a healthcare practitioner, one of the keys to treatment is recognizing that many people with FMS also do in fact have adrenal fatigue. Evaluating and treating this is likely an essential component in treating FMS.

Reviewing rheumatoid arthritis

Rheumatoid arthritis (RA) is a debilitating inflammatory arthritis that typically occurs in middle-aged individuals, but it can occur in people as young as their 20s and 30s. This deforming type of arthritis needs to be actively treated because, when full blown, it causes erosion of the joints.

An article published in 2008 in the medical journal *Best Practice and Research: Clinical Rheumatology* reviewed the interactions of the endocrine system, the nervous system, and inflammation with respect to the development of arthritis. With respect to the adrenal glands, the article noted two important points:

✔ Rheumatoid arthritis is associated with a significant amount of chronic inflammation, which should lead to high levels of cortisol. However, the authors noted decreased production of cortisol, given the significant amount of inflammation present.

✔ The authors also noted that the hypothalamus and pituitary gland, both of which produce hormones that affect adrenal glands, also demonstrated reduced levels of functioning. (See Chapter 2 for details on how these organs interact with each other.)

If you've been diagnosed with rheumatoid arthritis or you strongly suspect that you have it, you may have experienced one or more of the following symptoms:

✔ **Morning stiffness lasting for more than one hour:** This stiffness is dramatically different from just being a little stiff in the morning. This is a prolonged stiffness in many joints that can take over an hour to loosen up.

✔ **Arthritis that is bilateral and symmetric (affecting both sides of the body equally):** Common areas affected include the hands, especially the fingers.

✔ **Characteristic findings on X-rays:** Your healthcare provider can order X-rays to confirm the presence of rheumatoid arthritis. Examples of typical radiographic findings include narrowing of the joint spaces and erosion of the joints themselves.

✔ **Characteristic lab findings:** Your healthcare provider can order certain blood tests to aid in the diagnosis of rheumatoid arthritis. In rheumatoid arthritis, you may see an elevated sed rate (as you read in Chapter 5). Other labs that can be elevated include a rheumatoid factor as well as a specific antibody for rheumatoid arthritis alone called the *anti-cyclic citrullinated peptide* (or *anti-CCP*) antibody.

The traditional treatment for rheumatoid arthritis involves medications that suppress the immune system as a means of stopping the inflammation and joint swelling. These medications can include prednisone, methotrexate, and/or biologic agents, such as adalimumab (Humira). Alternative options for the treatment of rheumatoid arthritis include tart cherry extract (cherries are a potent natural inflammatory) and natural anti-inflammatory agents such as turmeric and bromelain. Please refer to Chapter 11, which reviews alternative remedies and treatments.

Looking at lupus

Systemic lupus erythematosus (SLE), more commonly known as just *lupus,* is an autoimmune disease commonly found in women in their late 30s to early 50s. This condition can affect multiple organs, including the heart, kidneys, joints, and lungs.

The cause of SLE isn't known; however, because it's an autoimmune disease, it involves the formation of *auto-antibodies* — antibodies that attack the person. That's why you may hear that in SLE, the body is literally attacking itself.

If you have lupus, you may have experienced one or more of the following symptoms:

- A butterfly rash on your face
- Photosensitivity (the sun really, really bothers you when you go outside)
- Ulcers in your mouth
- Heart problems: Lupus can affect the valves and cause *endocarditis* (inflammation of the heart valves) in a minority of patients; lupus can also cause inflammation of the *pericardium,* which is the outer aspect of the heart
- Kidneys problems and blood in the urine, protein in the urine, and/or acute kidney failure
- Positive blood (antibody) tests including a positive anti-nuclear antibody (ANA) and anti-double stranded DNA (anti-dsDNA)

The treatment of lupus may include prednisone, hydroxychloroquine (Plaquenil), methotrexate, and even stronger medication to suppress the immune system. Alternative treatment options for lupus include many options that appear earlier in this chapter. Before you begin using any alternative complementary treatments for lupus and rheumatoid arthritis, it's important that you speak with your healthcare practitioner. Lupus and RA are very potent inflammatory syndromes that require a personalized approach when considering the use of both traditional and alternative treatments. (For details on alternative remedies and treatments, see Chapter 11.)

Talking about thyroid dysfunction

The thyroid gland, which is located right below your voice box, produces the hormones thyroxine (also called T4) and triiodothyronine (T3). These hormones regulate body temperature; they're also intricately responsible for how well your cells do their jobs, including their chemical reactions and interactions with other cells. How well the cells and organs in your body perform these functions is referred to as the body's *metabolic rate*. Regulation of the body's metabolism maintains the integrity of your cells, tissues, and body systems.

Graves' disease, which is an autoimmune condition, is the most common cause of *hyperthyroidism* (an overactive thyroid). *Hypothyroidism* (an underactive thyroid) is much more prevalent in the United States than hyperthyroidism. Hypothyroidism is very common in women in their 30s and 40s, and the most common cause is an autoimmune condition called Hashimoto's thyroiditis.

Being diagnosed with Hashimoto's thyroiditis dramatically increases your risk of developing other autoimmune conditions. In 2010, the *American Journal of Medicine* reported the results of a questionnaire that looked at several hundred patients diagnosed with either Graves' disease or Hashimoto's thyroiditis. Researchers found that approximately 10 percent of those diagnosed with Graves' disease had another autoimmune condition. Among the patients diagnosed with Hashimoto's thyroiditis, approximately 14 percent had another autoimmune condition. The most frequently reported condition in this study was rheumatoid arthritis. Other conditions seen with increasing frequency included lupus; pernicious anemia, an autoimmune cause of B_{12} deficiency; vitiligo, an autoimmune condition affecting the skin; celiac disease; and Addison's disease, an autoimmune condition that can cause your adrenal glands to fail abruptly — think of it as adrenal shock requiring life-saving administration of steroids intravenously.

Here are symptoms of hyperthyroidism and hypothyroidism:

- ✔ **Hyperthyroidism:** A thyroid gland that's overactive or hyperfunctioning (producing too much thyroid hormone) can lead to high body temperatures, fast heart rate, diarrhea, intolerance to heat, and heart issues, including cardiac arrhythmias.

- ✔ **Hypothyroidism:** A thyroid gland that's underactive or producing too little thyroid hormone can produce symptoms of low body temperature, intolerance to cold, weight gain, fatigue, and lethargy.

Because the thyroid produces hormones, it's part of the body's endocrine system. A thyroid gland that isn't working well can affect the other organs that it interacts with, namely the hypothalamus, pituitary gland, and the adrenal glands.

The traditional treatments for hyperthyroidism include the use of beta blockers to decrease some of the symptoms of hyperthyroidism as well as medications such as propylthiouracil (PTU), which decreases the production of thyroid hormone. Depending on the cause of hyperthyroidism (there are several), an endocrinologist may order a special radioactive iodine test; this form of iodine can destroy thyroid tissue.

The traditional treatments for hypothyroidism include the prescription medication levothyroxine (Synthroid). However, you should be aware that there are other treatment options. One example is the use of another form of thyroid hormone called Armour Thyroid, which has higher amount of T3 compared to T4. The inclusion of iodine and trace minerals, including selenium, is important for supporting thyroid function. Be sure to speak with your healthcare practitioner to find out whether another option would be right for you. (For details about alternative remedies and treatments, check out Chapter 11.)

Digging into Lyme disease

Lyme disease is an infection, a tick-borne illness that causes chronic pain and disability in some people. It's transmitted by the deer tick, and the organism responsible for the condition is the bacterium *Borrelia burgdorferi*. If you live, work, or travel near woods or a forest area, then you're at higher risk of developing Lyme disease.

Lyme disease can affect multiple areas of the body, and many of the symptoms, including joint pain, stiffness, fatigue, and weakness, let Lyme disease mimic many other conditions. About 10 percent of people who develop Lyme disease get a characteristic bull's-eye skin rash, called *erythema chronicum migrans*. This rash is the most common initial manifestation of Lyme disease; it usually appears a few days after someone develops the condition, although in some people, the rash takes a few weeks to appear.

Untreated Lyme disease can be debilitating and disabling and can affect other organs of the body in addition to the joints. It can cause meningitis and *carditis,* or inflammation of the heart. Lyme disease is thought to be an underlying cause of fibromyalgia syndrome and chronic fatigue syndrome (see the earlier section "Fighting fibromyalgia syndrome").

The diagnosis of Lyme disease is confirmed via blood tests. The ELISA test is first, and the confirmatory test is the Western blot. Both of these tests need to be positive to confirm the diagnosis of Lyme disease, because many other inflammatory processes and chronic illnesses, such as rheumatoid arthritis and lupus, can cause the ELISA test to be falsely positive. Some healthcare practitioners use specialty labs (such as IGeneX) to confirm a diagnosis of Lyme disease.

Early in the course of the illness, the blood tests used to diagnose Lyme disease may not be positive. If the tests come back negative, they need to be repeated, especially if you've experienced a tick bite and strongly suspect that you have Lyme disease.

The treatment for Lyme disease is taking an antibiotic, doxycycline, twice a day for 21 days. In places where Lyme disease is epidemic, sometimes patients need to take antibiotics for a longer duration, especially if Lyme disease wasn't diagnosed initially.

That being said, you can do other things naturally to support your body, strengthen your immune system, and provide nutritional support; read about them in Chapter 11.

Understanding Acidosis and Its Link to Adrenal Fatigue

One of the biggest causes of and contributors to adrenal fatigue is acidosis. What exactly is acidosis? In the following sections, we define acidosis and pH, and we discuss what the body does to maintain a proper acid-base balance in the blood.

Explaining pH and acidosis

The human body exists in a normal acid-base balance, and pH is the way to measure how acidic or alkaline your body is (see Chapter 5 for details on measuring pH). The pH is a way of measuring the concentration of hydrogen ions (H^+) in the body.

Where do these ions come from? On a daily basis, the body breaks down the acid in the food you eat (especially protein) to produce these H^+ ions. They're eliminated by the kidneys, with the help of the adrenal glands. High acidity increases the workload of the kidneys and the adrenal glands to eliminate the excess H^+ ions. (See the next section for more about these organs' response to too much acid.)

In *acidosis,* the blood is too acidic. (The pH scale runs from 0 to 14, and a normal blood pH is 7.35 to 7.36. Lower than this level means that the blood is acidic, and higher means that the blood is alkaline.) The higher the number of hydrogen ions in the blood, the higher the blood's acidity and the lower the pH.

If your body is on the acidic side, you're at increased risk of developing a whole of host of problems, including chronic inflammation, pain, cancer, heart disease, and other chronic illnesses. A lower pH than normal increases the risk of developing malignancy, adrenal fatigue, osteoporosis, and kidney disease. Maintaining an acidic pH also dramatically contributes to the aging process.

Buffering excess acid

Every day, your body is under a constant barrage of acidity. From stress and an acid-forming diet based on the processed foods that you eat to the disease states that promote acidosis, your body struggles to maintain a normal acid-base balance.

Picture a seesaw with a bucket of acid on one end and a bucket of baking soda on the other end. If you were to look at a typical person in an industrialized society, you'd see the seesaw tip toward the side with the bucket of acid. So how does pH balance happen in the body? This occurs through the use of buffers and the work of organs, including the liver, kidneys, and adrenal glands.

Think of a buffer as a built-in safety mechanism that your body uses to maintain a normal pH balance. In response to an acid load, the body produces buffers in your cells, in the bloodstream, and in your bones. Examples of buffers in the bone include minerals such as calcium and magnesium. The calcium and magnesium are leached out of the bone as the body tries to maintain a normal acid-base balance. Over time, this leaching of calcium and magnesium can cause a thinning of the bone and contribute to osteoporosis.

In addition to buffers, certain organs of the body, namely the liver, kidneys, and adrenal glands, work hard to maintain pH balance. Here's how:

- **Liver:** Your liver is responsible for converting acid back into sodium bicarbonate (baking soda) through a chemical reaction.

- **Kidneys:** The kidneys, in concert with the adrenal glands, are responsible for eliminating the excess acid that's built up in the body each day.

  The kidneys also have a role in regenerating sodium bicarbonate; in fact, about 20 percent of the body's bicarbonate is generated in the kidneys. The serum bicarbonate level in the blood is used to provide a preliminary indication of the acid-base balance of the body. A level less than 22 milliequivalents per liter (mEq/L) can indicate that acidosis is present.

- **Adrenal glands:** To help the kidneys eliminate an acid load, the adrenal glands secrete a hormone called aldosterone.

Because the adrenal glands secrete aldosterone in response to acidosis, acidosis increases stress on the adrenal glands. In turn, adrenal fatigue can increase acidity; as the adrenal glands become less able to produce aldosterone, the kidneys may not be as able to eliminate the acid load.

Over time, acidosis can affect the integrity of the cells and change the environment of the cells from a normal state to an oxidative state. This causes the formation of free radicals, which promote the inflammatory process (see the earlier section "Understanding a normal inflammatory response"). In the next section, you find out about acidic conditions that really promote the inflammatory process.

Checking Out Common Causes of Acidosis

Many factors go into maintaining pH balance in the body. In this section, we go over some of the most common causes of acidosis, which increases your risk of developing adrenal fatigue. Some of these are dietary factors; others relate to problems with the organs themselves.

The Western diet

One contributor to acidosis is the Western or standard American diet. This diet is high in animal protein, which can promote oxidative stress. It's high in omega-6 fatty acids and low in omega-3 fatty acids — levels that can promote inflammation. The diet is also high in sugar, processed salt, chemicals, preservatives, and pesticides and toxins from the environment. The daily exposure to poor diet and toxins that deprive cells of the nutrients they need contributes to the development of acidic blood.

Certain food substances have a very high acid content and should be avoided if possible:

- Phosphoric acid is in many foods and beverages, including processed meats and carbonated beverages, namely sodas. The high acid load causes increased stress on the kidneys and the adrenal glands. A few studies suggest that continued phosphoric acid exposure over time can contribute to kidney disease.

- High fructose corn syrup and similar sugars are in many processed foods and beverages. These sugars have been shown to elevate blood pressure, cause weight gain, increase insulin levels, and cause insulin resistance as well as metabolic syndrome.

Changing your way of eating is fundamental to changing your health. Did you know that many vegetables are actually alkaline in nature? These include spinach, broccoli, asparagus, kale, and onions. In addition, many citrus fruits, such as lemons and oranges, have an alkaline effect on the body after they're digested and metabolized.

Diabetes

You're likely familiar with diabetes as a condition that involves high blood glucose levels. In *Type I diabetes mellitus,* the body simply doesn't make insulin. In *Type II diabetes mellitus,* the insulin has trouble getting into the cells in response to high blood glucose. One of the most common causes of Type II diabetes is obesity.

Watching your uric acid level

One of the most important blood tests that your healthcare provider can order is a uric acid level. *Uric acid* is a byproduct of cellular metabolism in the body. An elevated level can be a sign of significant underlying chronic illness. A high uric acid level can also mean that your cells are lacking key nutrients or are oxygen-deprived. In the setting of oxygen deprivation, the cells can become damaged. Increased oxidative stress and free-radical formation in the cell can increase the formation of uric acid. High uric acid levels (also called *hyperuricemia*) can indicate increased total body inflammation and acidosis.

Gout is a common medical condition that's caused by elevated uric acid levels. The uric acid in the blood can also be a source of debilitating arthritis, affecting the foot (often the big toe), the knee, and other joints in the body.

Elevated uric acid levels may indicate the health of your cells. Patients with congestive heart failure (CHF) with elevated uric acid levels actually have a worse prognosis. Treating these patients with medications that lower uric acid levels in the bloodstream may increase their longevity and quality of life and portend a favorable prognosis. Patients with diabetes can have an elevated uric acid level as well.

The body converts diets high in animal protein to uric acid. One of the basic treatments for an elevated uric level is an alkaline-based diet. If you're able to alkalinize your urine, uric acid is soluble and is easier for the kidneys to eliminate.

Diabetes mellitus can cause eye disease *(retinopathy),* affect the integrity of the nerves and nervous system *(neuropathy),* and cause kidney disease. In fact, diabetes is the leading cause of kidney disease in the U.S. (See the next section for info on kidney disease.)

From an acid-base perspective, diabetes mellitus is an acid-producing state. Diabetes can cause acidosis for a couple of reasons:

- ✔ When the blood sugar levels are high, the body can generate a type of acid called a *ketoacid.* Diabetic ketoacidosis is a condition that often requires admission to the hospital and intravenous insulin.

- ✔ Diabetes can cause a type of acidosis by affecting the kidneys' ability to eliminate excess acid in the urine. A few studies suggest that the acid-producing effects of diabetes are enough to increase the formation of kidney stones, especially uric acid stones.

Diabetes can produce *advanced glycosylated end products (AGEs).* AGEs are significant promoters of the inflammatory response that we describe earlier in this chapter.

If you have diabetes, one of the most highly recommended dietary plans is the low-glycemic diet. To understand this diet, you need to be familiar with the *glycemic index,* which is a measure of a food substance's ability to increase the insulin response after you consume that food. Candy and other foods high in sugar have a high glycemic index because they stimulate an increased insulin response. Certain fruits like bananas also have a high glycemic index, whereas others, such as apples, have a lower glycemic index.

In general, a plant-based diet is low on the glycemic index. A strict alkaline-based diet can help restore pH balance to the body and, as a bonus, help you lose weight and lower your blood glucose levels.

For more information on the glycemic index, check out *Glycemic Index Diet For Dummies* by Meri Raffetto, RD; *Glycemic Index Cookbook For Dummies* by Meri Raffetto, RD, and Rosanne Rust, MS, RD, LDN; and *Diabetes For Dummies* by Alan L. Rubin, MD (all published by Wiley).

Kidney disease

The kidneys and the adrenal glands play an important role in eliminating excess acid from the body. Diseased kidneys, especially in the latter stages of kidney disease, have difficulty eliminating the excess acid from the body, which leads to acidosis. Diabetes is the leading cause of kidney disease, so you can run into a real problem if you have both conditions. Other causes of kidney disease include hypertension, genetic causes such as polycystic kidney disease, and various types of inflammatory conditions called *nephritis.* Examples include medication-induced nephritis and lupus-induced nephritis.

Symptoms of kidney disease can include swelling of the legs, the presence of blood in the urine, urine that may be frothy or bubbly, and high blood pressure that's difficult to control. Many times, however, a person doesn't have any symptoms. The only indication that a kidney problem is present is through abnormalities on the blood work (an elevated creatinine level) or the presence of blood or protein in the urine. If you have a history of hypertension or diabetes (the two most common causes of kidney disease), ask your doctor or healthcare practitioner about the status of your kidney function.

Advanced kidney disease certainly affects the body's ability to get rid of excess acid. The corollary to this is also true: Several studies suggest that acidosis has the potential to worsen kidney disease. Not only can alkali supplementation improve bone health, but it may also prevent kidney disease from worsening.

Here are several things you can to do improve your kidney health:

- Eat a plant-based diet.
- Take a daily probiotic.
- Drink alkaline water.
- Supplement with vitamin D if your vitamin D levels are low in the blood (refer to Chapter 11).
- If you have diabetes and/or high blood pressure, get your blood glucose levels and blood pressure levels under control.

Please refer to Chapter 20 for more information on improving kidney function. By optimizing kidney function, you can help eliminate acidosis and correct the pH of the blood.

Lung disease

Together, two types of lung disease, emphysema and chronic bronchitis, remain the most common reason besides congestive heart failure (CHF) for admission to the hospital. Many people are also suffering from sleep apnea and a technical condition called *alveolar hypoventilation;* simply stated, they're having breathing problems, especially with eliminating carbon dioxide from the lungs.

Normally, every time you breathe, you inhale oxygen, which goes deep into your lungs. The alveoli in the lungs avidly take in the oxygen, and then you exhale carbon dioxide. If you have lung disease, you may not be fully able to get rid of the excess carbon dioxide, so the acid level builds up in the blood and causes acidosis.

If the lungs are unable to eliminate the carbon dioxide, then the kidneys and the adrenal glands have to work that much harder to eliminate the acid load from the body. Medical conditions that affect the lung also increase total body inflammation, which is a further stressor on the adrenal glands.

The two biggest reasons for lung issues in the U.S. are cigarette smoking and obesity. Here are some things you can do to improve your lung health:

- Stop smoking.
- At home and in the workplace, be aware of and minimize exposures to toxic substances such as asbestos and heavy metals.

✔ Take a probiotic. Taking a daily probiotic has been shown to decrease the severity of lung problems such as asthma.

✔ Increase your omega-3 fatty acid intake; it may have an anti-inflammatory effect.

Please refer to Chapter 20 for more ways to optimize lung function.

Chapter 8

Nutrition's Role in Adrenal Fatigue

*P*oor nutrition is a huge contributor to the development of adrenal fatigue. The effects of vitamin and mineral deficiencies and poor intestinal health can exhaust already-fatigued adrenal glands. These abnormalities aren't just causes of adrenal fatigue; they can also worsen inflammation, make you more susceptible to infection, and increase your risk of developing autoimmune disease.

This chapter gives you the lowdown on the link between adrenal fatigue and intestinal health/micronutrient deficiencies. Attending to these factors is essential in restoring adrenal gland function.

Surveying the Small Intestine's Structure

We believe that adrenal fatigue can be both a cause and a consequence of the body's organ systems being out of kilter. The root of all chronic illness and inflammation is in the small intestine, which does a heck of a lot more than just process and absorb food.

Picture your small intestine as a long, winding tube that connects to the stomach. The small intestine absorbs nutrients and passes the residual food waste to the large intestine, which is responsible for eliminating the waste as stools.

If you look at a close-up picture of a small intestine, you'll see cells that fit tightly together to maximize the absorption of nutrients. The cells are attached to one another by fasteners called *tight junctions*. They're important for maintaining the integrity of the intestine, and they act as the glue that keeps all the cells in working order. In fact, one of the hallmarks of intestinal dysfunction (see the next section) is the loss of the tight junctions. Figure 8-1 compares healthy intestinal cells to damaged intestinal cells.

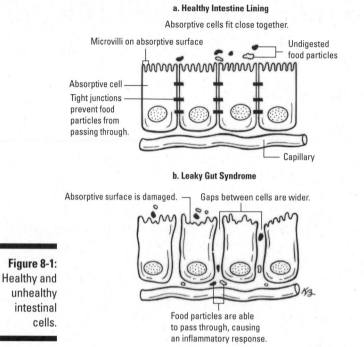

a. Healthy Intestine Lining

Absorptive cells fit close together.

Microvilli on absorptive surface

Undigested food particles

Absorptive cell

Tight junctions prevent food particles from passing through.

Capillary

b. Leaky Gut Syndrome

Absorptive surface is damaged.

Gaps between cells are wider.

Figure 8-1:
Healthy and unhealthy intestinal cells.

Food particles are able to pass through, causing an inflammatory response.

Illustration by Kathryn Born, MA

Picture now that your intestine is an ecosystem filled with trillions — yes, trillions — of bacteria (and other tiny organisms) called *microflora.* The delicate balance of this intestinal ecosystem is the foundation of all health. The opposite is also true: An imbalance in this ecosystem is a major contributing factor to chronic illness and inflammation.

Your intestine is home to good bacteria and bad bacteria. The good bacteria outnumber the bad bacteria and keep them at bay. Bad things can happen if the bad bacteria get control of the intestine. The good bacteria include those in the *Lactobacillus* genus, such as *Lactobacillus acidophilus.* Another important genus is *Bifidobacterium.* And there's also the species *Streptococcus thermophilus* (this species differs from the bad *Streptococcus,* which is pathogenic). Examples of bad intestinal bacteria include the infamous *E. coli* and *Clostridium difficile.*

The good bacteria have many beneficial functions, including

✔ Helping in the absorption of nutrients

✔ Synthesizing vitamins, including vitamin K

✔ Modulating immune system function

The intestine has a layer called the *mucosa,* which comes in direct contact with digested food. The mucosa is the first defense against infections, especially bacterial infections. Good intestinal microflora can help stimulate the production of certain antibodies called *immunoglobulins.* A good example is IgA, which is important in protecting this mucosal layer from destructive bacteria. Research suggests that good microflora also help bind infectious agents to the intestinal mucous. They're then consumed, or *phagocytized,* and eradicated by other immune cells in the small intestine.

Being breastfed is important in the development of an infant's immune system. Breast milk contains *prebiotics,* which cause the good microflora that are already present in the intestine to create more good microflora. When it comes to helping develop a healthy immune system in a newborn infant, breastfeeding is the way to go.

Investigating Intestinal Dysbiosis

Intestinal dysbiosis is a general term that refers to an unhealthy small intestine due to an imbalance in gastrointestinal bacteria. You see the loss of the integrity of the intestinal cells in Figure 8-1 (see the preceding section); the tight junctions are worn down, and gaps exist between the cells. The cells have lost the glue that keeps them working well.

Any one of these factors can cause changes in your intestinal microflora, though several are often present at the same time:

✔ Stress (both physical and psychological; see Chapter 6)

✔ Chronic illness

✔ Antibiotics and other medication use

✔ *Candida* overgrowth

✔ Processed foods and the Western or standard American diet

✔ Exposures to trigger foods and lectins

Making the gut-brain connection

Compared to 10 years ago, depression, anxiety, dementia, and autism have markedly increased in incidence. The focus of mental health therapy used to be on medications that targeted specific areas of the brain (that is, selective serotonin uptake inhibitors, or SSRIs, such as fluoxetine [Prozac]). New research is focusing on how the health of the intestine can affect the health of the brain.

Normalizing intestinal flora and replacing key micronutrients are part of a new focus in treating mental health conditions. For example, normalizing intestinal health may be crucial in the treatment of depression and other medical conditions, including dementia.

The bacterial flora of the intestine does much more than digest food. Not only do these bacteria reduce inflammation, but they may also alter brain chemistry. More research is being done in this area, but the implication is clear: Normalization of intestinal microflora likely has an important role in the management of these conditions.

The symptoms of intestinal dysbiosis often depend on the cause of the dysbiosis as well as how unhealthy the small intestine is. Common symptoms that should clue you in are

- Bloating and abdominal distention
- Flatulence
- Nausea and/or vomiting
- Diarrhea and/or constipation

Untreated intestinal dysbiosis has a ripple effect on the entire body. Different people are affected in different ways, but here are some general consequences of an unhealthy bowel:

- Worsening chronic illness
- Systemic inflammation (see Chapter 7)
- Malnutrition (we talk about nutritional deficiencies later in this chapter)
- Cancer
- Adrenal fatigue and adrenal exhaustion

Intestinal dysbiosis increases total body inflammation, which causes the development of adrenal fatigue. It increases the likelihood of developing chronic illness, and it can worsen the severity and symptoms of a chronic illness that's already present. Dysbiosis also affects the ability of the small intestine to effectively absorb vitamins, minerals, and micronutrients that are necessary for adrenal gland functioning. Nutrient depletion is a direct cause of adrenal fatigue.

This section discusses some of the major contributors to the development of intestinal dysbiosis.

Assessing antibiotic use

Antibiotics can really disrupt the delicate balance of the intestinal ecosystem, killing off the good bacteria that keep the bad bacteria at bay. Even one dose of an antibiotic can have a significant effect on the ecosystem of the intestine.

Unfortunately, healthcare practitioners prescribe huge amounts of antibiotics. Most people expect that they'll get an antibiotic when they see their doctors, and some parents practically demand that their children receive antibiotics regardless of whether they're warranted. The medical profession is just starting to realize the negative effects of the overuse of antibiotics.

Be aware of some of the clinical consequences of antibiotic use:

- **Diarrhea:** Antibiotics can cause diarrhea, a condition called *antibiotic associated colitis.* Luckily, this can resolve when you stop using the antibiotic.

- ***Clostridium difficile* colitis:** See the nearby sidebar for details on this inflammatory condition.

- **Yeast overgrowth:** We discuss this significant side effect in the next section.

Some really bad bugs: *Clostridium difficile* colitis

Imbalance in your intestinal ecosystem can contribute to the development of some really bad medical conditions, such as *Clostridium difficile (C. diff)* colitis. This potentially fatal condition is the one of the most common causes of hospital-acquired infections.

C. diff is a natural part of your intestinal ecosystem, kept in check by the presence of the good intestinal bacteria. However, rampant use of antibiotics and certain other medications (for example, proton pump inhibitors) can cause these bad bacteria to flourish in the intestine.

(Other risk factors include advanced age and poor nutrition.)

A proliferation of *C. diff* in the intestine can have devastating consequences, including a really bad *colitis* (inflammation of the colon). Complications of this form of colitis can cause intestinal perforation that may require emergency surgery; they can also include acute kidney failure and multiorgan system failure. Even with aggressive treatment, the mortality rate is high. Awareness is the key to preventing this condition.

Which antibiotics do you need to be aware of? Well, any class of antibiotics has the propensity to alter the intestinal flora, but certain classes — including the penicillins, cephalosporins, fluoroquinolones, and clindamycin — have been recognized as causes of antibiotic associated colitis and *Clostridium difficile* colitis.

Think of your immune system as a part of you that matures and develops as you do. You can avoid damaging it by minimizing antibiotic use. Of course, we're not saying that a patient shouldn't be prescribed an antibiotic when absolutely needed, but be cautious, especially with children. The next time an antibiotic is a treatment option, both you and your practitioner need to ask, "Is this antibiotic really necessary? Would a natural remedy work to boost the immune system and help fight off that infection?" (See Chapter 11 for information on these types of remedies.) If an antibiotic is truly the best treatment, ask whether you can take *probiotics* (beneficial microorganisms) with it to help replenish the good bacteria. This helps minimize the degree of damage that the antibiotic does to the intestinal tract.

Considering Candida: A fungus among us

Bacteria aren't the only organisms in the intestinal ecosystem. *Candida,* the most common genus of yeast (a fungus), is also in your small intestine. It's usually present in very small amounts, and the beneficial bacterial flora help keep the level of *Candida* in check.

Overgrowth of *Candida* in the intestine is a problem largely unrecognized in the United States. The factors contributing to the overgrowth of *Candida* are

- ✔ The overuse of antibiotics (see the preceding section)
- ✔ A Western diet, an acidic diet, and or a diet high in sugar (see the next section)
- ✔ Stress
- ✔ Chronic illness and malnutrition
- ✔ Diabetes mellitus (a significant risk factor)

The symptoms of *Candida* overgrowth (and how to reverse them) can include the following:

- ✔ **Weakness/fatigue:** One of the main symptoms of *Candida* overgrowth is weakness and fatigue that simply doesn't get better and persists for a long time. The key to treating this is recognizing the symptom early on in conjunction with the other symptoms listed in this section.

✔ **Flu-like symptoms, including arthralgias (joint pains) and myalgias (muscle pains) that can persist and even worsen over time:** Many things can cause leaking of tight cell-to-cell junctions (refer to Figure 8-1 earlier in the chapter), and *Candida* is one of them. *Candida* can secrete fungal toxins called *mycotoxins* that can leak out into the bloodstream and have systemic effects, including joint pain and flu-like symptoms. The common recommendation from modern practitioners? Avoid foods that are high in sugar.

✔ **Fungal skin rashes:** The presence of skin rashes that don't go away, along with recurrent yeast infections, can be connected with *Candida* overgrowth syndrome. How do you know if you have a fungal skin rash? Well, general characteristics of fungal skin infections are skin lesions that are scaly, red, and really itchy. Usually they're present on a certain area of the body, as in athlete's foot. They can also occur on the chest, the arms, or the legs.

The short-term treatment of this condition includes topical antifungal medications such as clotrimazole (Lotrimin). Your healthcare practitioner may also prescribe a medication that treats fungal infections, a common example being fluconazole (Diflucan). The long-term treatment is the use of natural antifungal agents, including garlic and olive leaf (see Chapter 11), as well as eliminating sugar from your diet.

✔ **Weight gain:** Maybe you've decreased your caloric intake and are exercising more (congratulations!), but you're still having a hard time losing weight. Maybe you're even gaining weight. If so, suspect *Candida* overgrowth. Simply put, if you don't eliminate the yeast overgrowth in the intestine, losing weight will be difficult, if not impossible. Chapter 11 points out that one of the keys to combating fungal overgrowth is restricting sugar intake.

✔ **Abdominal bloating:** Fungal overgrowth in the intestine can cause bloating and distention. Yeast rises, especially when your diet contains excess sugar. That's why you can end up with an abdomen that looks like a giant loaf of bread.

Digging into the standard American diet

Your diet is probably very SAD. The Western or *standard American diet (SAD)* consists of food that is processed, pro-inflammatory, acidic, high in calories, and of little nutritional value. The diet contributes to the overgrowth of bad microflora in the intestine. That's a formula for health problems. The American diet is a significant contributor to many of the nation's health problems.

Taking care of your gut if you have kidney disease

About 31 million people in the United States have kidney disease (about one in every eight to ten individuals). Diabetes and hypertension represent the top two causes of kidney disease; because so many people have these conditions, chronic kidney disease (CKD) is fairly widespread.

The role of the kidneys is to filter and eliminate the toxins that build up in the body each day. Some research suggests that these toxins can accumulate in the bowel, altering the intestinal microflora and contributing to the loss of bowel integrity. Here's a common example: Mr. X has diabetes, and blood work demonstrates the presence of kidney disease. His diabetes is uncontrolled, so his high blood glucose levels are causing increased stress on his adrenal glands. The diabetes also contributes to a *Candida* overgrowth, which is affecting the microflora. Add to this scenario his likely prior antibiotic use, which has also altered his intestinal microflora, and

Mr. X has what's known as a *leaky gut*. In the setting of kidney disease, the uremic toxins can collect in the bowel, further damaging the intestinal microflora.

If you're diagnosed with kidney disease, you need to have a long discussion with your healthcare provider. Part of this discussion must include how to keep your intestinal microflora healthy. Why? For anyone with kidney disease, the presence of uremic toxins in the bowel increases total body inflammation. That's bad. The increased inflammation not only increases adrenal stress but also can worsen kidney disease over time.

A special type of probiotic can help eliminate the uremic toxins from the intestine. If you have kidney disease, speak with your kidney doctor about whether probiotics are appropriate in your situation.

What are the nutritional guidelines you should follow? Most folks remember the Food Pyramid, but it underwent a few revisions, especially in light of health problems plaguing the United States. Here are the highlights of the new and revised guidelines (now known as MyPlate, published by the United States Department of Agriculture; see www.choosemyplate.gov):

✔ Restrict sugar, fats, and the majority of oils. Note that the type of fat matters. You want to be sure that about a fifth of your diet includes foods that contain healthy fats. Bad fats include trans fats and saturated fats. Good fats are in foods high in polyunsaturated fatty acids; examples include fish (such as salmon and trout) and nuts and seeds (such as sunflower seeds).

✔ Increase fruit and vegetable intake — especially vegetables. Your goal should be to eat 2.5 to 5 cups of vegetables and 1.5 to 4 cups of fruit each day.

BPA: Using caution with cans

Before you pick up your favorite can of tomatoes, be sure you see "BPA-free" on the label. BPA, or *bisphenol A,* is found in plastics and resins. The food industry may consider BPA to be safe, but studies are beginning to show an adverse relationship between BPA and fertility, the prostate gland, and brain development. Hence, many people — both health practitioners and the public — are concerned about plastic bottles, canned foods (particularly acidic canned foods), and food storage containers.

Good news! You can now find BPA-free water bottles, canned foods, and storage containers. To be safe, look for items stored in glass jars over canned and don't use plastic food storage and service items.

✔ Stay away from juices that are high in sugar. The sugar content negates any health benefit the juice may provide. Remember that sugar increases total body inflammation exponentially; it's also fuel for *Candida* (see the preceding section for info on *Candida* overgrowth).

Combine fresh fruits and vegetables to make your own juice. See Chapter 14 for info on juicers and some great fruit-and-veggie combinations.

✔ Limit dairy unless the product is fermented, such as yogurt and kefir.

✔ Increase your consumption of foods that are not refined or processed.

✔ If you eat animal protein, go for fish and lean meats.

People who change their diets often experience vast improvements in health. And you can experiment, too. We suggest you consult a holistic doctor or a registered dietitian (RD) for any major diet changes.

Fighting food sensitivities and food allergies

Some foods you consume can trigger an inflammatory reaction; that's how your body reacts to the food. In this section, we talk about trigger foods and discuss lectins and food sensitivities.

Contrasting food sensitivities and food allergies

A *food sensitivity* is an inflammatory/immune reaction your body has to the lectins in a food. *Lectins* are proteins found in many foods, especially grains and nuts. The lectins in your particular *trigger food* set off an immune reaction in the intestine. It can cause leaking of the tight junctions of the small intestine cells and lead to leaky gut syndrome (*increased intestinal permeability,* in doctor talk). The body views the lectins as foreign invaders and forms antibodies against them.

Common symptoms of food sensitivity include fatigue, muscle and/or joint aches, headaches, excessive flatulence, diarrhea, bloating, heartburn, confusion, and irritability. Often these symptoms occur several hours after the consumption of the offending food. If you say, "Must have been something I ate," chances are you're exactly right.

A food allergy, on the other hand, is quite different from a food sensitivity. A *food allergy* triggers an allergic reaction, not an inflammatory response. Common allergic symptoms include tongue swelling, watery eyes, wheezing, and acute shortness of breath. A food allergy can develop into a medical emergency. Whereas food sensitivity often occurs several hours after you eat the trigger food, food allergy symptoms often appear very quickly.

Particularly severe allergies can cause a major overreaction of the immune system. The result can be *anaphylaxis,* an emergency situation requiring immediate attention and treatment with epinephrine. Anaphylaxis is a serious allergic reaction that comes on rapidly and may cause death, likely through heart attack or its cousin, cardiac arrest.

Pinpointing trigger foods

Unless you identify and stop consuming the trigger food, the symptoms may persist. Common causes of food sensitivities include foods that contain lactose or gluten. Common causes of food allergies include eggs, nuts, wheat, fish, and shellfish. That being said, be aware that *any* food has the potential to be a trigger food, even fruits and vegetables.

Consider keeping a food diary in order to identify potential trigger foods. Each person is different, and different foods can trigger different reactions. If you find that you experience the symptoms of a food sensitivity or allergy, you can eliminate what you think may be the trigger food from your diet.

If the idea of a food diary is cumbersome or overwhelming, consider going the medical route and taking food sensitivity tests. ALCAT (www.ALCAT.com) and LEAP (Lifestyle Eating and Performance, www.nowleap.com) are the two most commonly used blood tests for looking at triggers from food, dyes, additives, and preservatives. Both companies provide practitioners who can assist you with understanding the results and creating a diet plan.

Confronting celiac disease

Celiac disease is an inflammatory autoimmune condition of the small intestine caused by *gluten,* which is a protein in wheat, rye, and barley. According to an article from the *American Journal of Gastroenterology* in 2012, approximately 1 in every 141 people is thought to have celiac disease. Our opinion is that celiac disease is more prevalent than that.

Your small intestine is where many of the nutrients from the foods you eat and the medications and supplements you take are absorbed. Celiac disease (officially, *gluten-sensitive enteropathy*) affects your intestine's ability to absorb these nutrients, creating a condition called *malabsorption.* The significant nutrient deficiencies that can result from this condition include low levels of iron; folate; vitamins B_{12}, C, and D; magnesium; and calcium. (We discuss these deficiencies later in this chapter.)

Believe it or not, diagnosing celiac disease can be difficult. Though many people report problems with nausea, abdominal bloating, flatulence, greasy stools, and/or weight loss, many others present with only extreme fatigue or weakness. Sometimes doctors find celiac disease only through elevated liver function from routine tests taken for something else entirely.

Although your healthcare provider can order certain blood tests to diagnose celiac disease, right now the best way to diagnose it is to obtain tissue from the small intestine, often through a biopsy. A gastroenterologist does this procedure with an endoscopy.

Treating celiac disease basically means avoiding anything with gluten in it, which is becoming easy to do. Some supermarkets and most natural food co-ops have dedicated gluten-free aisles, and some restaurants have gluten-free selections. The Internet is full of purveyors of gluten-free foods.

Be aware that gluten isn't only in bread products; it's also found in lots of other foods (including some you may not think of, such as soy sauce). Check out www.celiac.com for a list of some gluten-containing foods. Make sure that your nutritional supplements are gluten-free, too. Further, you may be surprised to know that certain household products have gluten in them. Look at your hair products, shampoos, skin lotions, or creams. Reading labels is important; you want to avoid anything that contains gluten even if you aren't putting the product in your mouth.

Don't panic! Having celiac disease doesn't mean you have to eliminate all grains from your diet. Grains and seeds such as quinoa, millet, and rice are gluten-free and delicious as well.

Navigating Nutrient Deficiencies

Nutrient deficiencies can affect multiple organ systems. In this section, we identify key nutrient deficiencies that affect adrenal health. We focus on important minerals (including magnesium, calcium, and potassium), trace minerals (including zinc, chromium, and selenium), and vitamins. Check out Chapter 11 for natural remedies that can help correct these deficiencies.

We can't underscore enough the importance of getting your intestinal tract on track (as described earlier in the chapter) before supplementing nutrients. If your gut is leaky, your intestine's ability to absorb these nutrients is compromised. Please refer to Chapter 11 for ways to improve your intestinal health and halt *Candida* overgrowth.

Managing magnesium

The mineral magnesium is part of the energy mechanism that keeps cells running smoothly. Magnesium is a catalyst for more than 200 chemical reactions in the human body. The energy centers in your cells, including those in the adrenal glands, need magnesium for optimal operation.

Magnesium is mainly found in your bones, so magnesium depletion can have detrimental effects on bone health. It can contribute to the development of osteoporosis. Low magnesium levels can also affect the absorption of other minerals, including potassium and calcium (which we discuss in the next section).

Eating whole foods for their nutrients

Nutrition is more than just nutrients; food can be satisfying and healing, too. Whole foods host undiscovered nutrients — a new world of *phytochemicals* (chemical compounds that occur naturally in plants). Nutrition is a relatively new science that's growing every day. New information is constantly emerging (remember when people thought eating eggs increased your cholesterol?), and nutrients are still being discovered.

What has remained consistent is where nutrients come from: food. And the most nutrient-dense options are whole foods (foods that aren't refined or processed) in their purest forms. An orange is more than just vitamin C; it boasts fiber and citrus bioflavonoids. Chia seeds provide fiber, protein, omega fatty acids, calcium, phosphorous, and manganese. Although scientists continue to try to isolate foods' phytochemicals to see how they work against cancer and disease, the results often show that the best disease-fighting and anti-cancer effects come from the whole food, not the isolated compound.

The moral of the story: Be open to new foods. Begin identifying areas where you can improve your diet, and take small steps toward healing. (Flip to Part IV for recipes that use whole foods in battling adrenal fatigue.)

Magnesium is crucial for maintaining muscle strength and endurance because it dilates blood vessels, improving blood flow to the muscles (which is important not only for muscle health but also for toxin removal). Very low magnesium levels can cause symptoms such as muscle spasm and muscle weakness. Some people also experience numbness and tingling in their extremities.

Low magnesium levels also increase total body inflammation and may be a significant contributing factor to fibromyalgia, migraine headaches, and diabetes.

One major cause of magnesium deficiency is the Western or standard American diet. Green vegetables, nuts, and seeds are all excellent sources of magnesium, but most people don't eat these foods on a regular basis. Another common reason for magnesium deficiency is intestinal dysbiosis, which can affect the absorption of magnesium. Note that a commonly prescribed class of medications called *diuretics,* which are used in the treatment of high blood pressure and edema, can also cause low magnesium levels. These medications increase the urinary excretion of magnesium.

The good news: Magnesium supplementation can decrease the frequency and intensity of migraine headaches; it can also lower blood pressure, improve blood vessel health, and decrease insulin resistance, which is the hallmark of Type II diabetes.

The most common way to know whether your magnesium levels are low is a simple blood test. However, be aware that the magnesium level measured in the blood may not accurately reflect the levels of magnesium in the cells. That being said, other tests used to measure magnesium can be more cumbersome, and some people question their reliability. So overall, the blood test is a better way to go.

On routine blood work, most normal reference ranges for magnesium are from 1.6 to 2.6 milligrams per deciliter (mg/dL). Note the significant difference between the values at the high and low ends of the range. Lower normal levels may represent a deficiency of magnesium within the cells. For me (coauthor Rich), the goal of treatment is to get the magnesium levels in the blood into the higher end of the normal range.

Looking at potassium and calcium

Potassium and calcium often work together with magnesium (covered in the preceding section). They're absorbed in the small intestine, and deficiencies of one of these minerals can affect the levels of the others.

Potassium is important for the health of your cells, especially in your nerves and heart. Very low or very high potassium levels can have detrimental effects on heart function. Calcium is important for heart and bone health. Like magnesium, calcium and potassium are important for the cells of the adrenal glands to function.

With the Western or standard American diet, potassium levels tend to be on the low side. The same is true for calcium. For most folks in Western society, these levels aren't low enough to cause symptoms. Fortunately, your health-care practitioner can order blood tests that tell you whether your potassium and calcium levels are low.

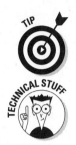

Green leafy vegetables are excellent sources of both potassium and calcium. Please refer to Chapter 11 for info on potassium and calcium supplementation.

When you go to see the doctor, your blood work will probably show that your calcium level is normal. What the tests won't indicate is that your body may be leaching calcium from your bones to maintain normal levels in the blood. Your body's natural tendency is to try to balance mineral levels in your blood whatever way it can. Plus, the modern diet is very acidic, and that acidity can serve as a stimulus for leaching calcium from bone.

Talking about trace minerals

The three trace minerals in this section — zinc, chromium, and selenium — are vital to total body and adrenal health. They're called *trace* minerals because you need to consume only small amounts of them. Even though only small amounts are needed, many people are deficient in them due to their diet. Replacement of these minerals is important; however, taking too much of any trace mineral can also adversely affect your health.

Zinc

Zinc is a micronutrient that's important for many cellular functions and cellular chemical reactions. Zinc has a role in maintaining a healthy immune system, too, and it's a necessary mineral for wound healing and adrenal function.

Many medical conditions can increase the likelihood of developing low zinc levels, including liver and kidney disease and chronic inflammation. Chronic inflammation can cause changes to the intestinal flora, leading to dysbiosis. The reverse is also true: Intestinal dybiosis can directly cause malabsorption as well as be a direct cause of inflammation. (See the earlier section "Investigating Intestinal Dysbiosis.")

Taking in enough zinc is important because the body doesn't naturally produce it. You can find out whether your zinc level is low through a blood or saliva test. Symptoms of very low zinc levels can include an unhealthy immune system (that is, increased difficulty fighting off infections), decreased appetite, diarrhea, and losing your hair.

Chromium

Chromium is an important micronutrient that has several functions, including aiding the cell's ability to handle glucose and insulin, helping your body process carbohydrates. Adrenal fatigue can be associated with both high and low blood glucose levels (see Chapter 4 for details). If you have adrenal fatigue, chromium is important in keeping your blood glucose at a normal level. A chromium deficiency is also considered to be a possible risk factor for developing diabetes and possibly heart disease (though the latter conclusion is more controversial).

Besides higher than normal blood glucose levels, symptoms of chromium deficiency can include increased weakness, muscle fatigue, anxiety, and increased irritability.

Chromium deficiency, like other trace mineral deficiencies, is often due to the Western or standard American diet. Healthcare practitioners opt to supplement this mineral after taking a thorough dietary history. Please refer to Chapter 11 for info on chromium supplementation.

Selenium

Selenium is an antioxidant that helps protect your cells from free-radical damage. This mineral is important for cell function as well as for maximizing thyroid and adrenal function. It has also been shown to have cancer-fighting effects.

Signs of selenium deficiency can include increased fatigue and increased weakness. Because selenium deficiency is closely tied to thyroid dysfunction, anyone who has been diagnosed with hypothyroidism is often felt to be selenium deficient. In women, selenium deficiency has been connected to reproductive disorders.

Eggs, nuts, and seeds are foods that are very high in selenium. For info on selenium supplementation, please refer to Chapter 11.

Breaking down the B vitamins

Deficiencies of B vitamins can affect your overall health. Many of the B vitamins are essential for optimal health, but a specific B vitamin, vitamin B_5 (pantothenic acid), is especially important for adrenal health. Here we examine some of the B vitamins you need to pay attention to when you're dealing with stress and adrenal fatigue.

Thiamine (vitamin B_1)

Vitamin B_1 (thiamine) is important for the cells to work efficiently and for adequate nerve and muscle function. It plays a role not only in how the cells produce energy but also in how your body processes glucose. Because high or low levels of glucose can cause issues in adrenal fatigue sufferers (as we describe in Chapter 4), vitamin B_1 deficiency is particularly troubling.

You may think of vitamin B_1 deficiency as something that occurs only in people who abuse alcohol; however, many people, especially those with chronic illnesses, may be deficient in this vitamin. If you've been in the hospital, especially in critical care, you're very likely to be low in vitamin B_1. If you're a dialysis patient or you're one of millions of people taking a class of medication called *diuretics* (also known as water pills), you're probably low in vitamin B_1.

A number of medical conditions are related to vitamin B_1 deficiency, and significant deficiencies of vitamin B_1 can affect heart function, perhaps leading to cardiac failure and death.

Severe deficiencies of vitamin B_1 can include a condition called *Wernicke's encephalopathy,* which includes acute confusion and difficulty walking. This condition is commonly seen in people with a history of alcoholism.

Note that many people have low levels of vitamin B_1 without having any acute symptoms. If your healthcare provider suspects you may be low in vitamin B_1, you can take a blood test. That being said, the test is usually unnecessary, and often your practitioner will talk with you about changing your diet or using supplementation (see Chapter 11 for details). Foods that are high in vitamin B_1 include fish, nuts, and seeds.

Riboflavin (vitamin B_2)

Vitamin B_2 (riboflavin) is important for the function of the *mitochondria* (the energy/power centers of the cell) and of the adrenal glands. Researchers believe that vitamin B_2 works with vitamin C, basically increasing the function of the cells in the adrenal glands. Vitamin B_2 is also key to maintaining a healthy nervous system.

Signs of severe B_2 deficiency can include weakness, sore throat, skin cracking (especially at the outer corners of the mouth), and a swollen tongue. The eyes can be especially affected; symptoms include blurry vision, double vision, and *photophobia* (sensitivity to light). Note that as with the other vitamins, levels that are simply lower than normal don't cause these symptoms.

Green vegetables, fish, and fortified cereals are excellent sources of vitamin B_2.

Niacin (vitamin B_3)

Niacin is a B vitamin that helps increase the levels of HDL (the good cholesterol). It's also important in adrenal gland functioning, acting as an essential ingredient in the production of adrenal hormones.

Significant depletion of niacin may cause a condition called *pellagra.* Symptoms of pellagra include the three *d*'s: dermatitis, diarrhea, and depression. However, lower-than-normal levels of this vitamin rarely cause any of these symptoms.

Foods high in vitamin B_3 include fish, poultry, and nuts.

Pantothenic acid (vitamin B₅)

Of all the B vitamins, vitamin B_5 (pantothenic acid) is possibly the most critical to adrenal gland function. Different lab-based studies have demonstrated that it can boost supplementation of adrenal hormones, including cortisol and progesterone. In addition, it can help regulate the response of the adrenal glands' receptors and prevent them from being so hyper-responsive. Without proper B_5 supplementation, a person with adrenal fatigue is at risk of developing adrenal exhaustion; the adrenal glands simply won't be able to meet the metabolic demands of the body. Like the other B vitamins, vitamin B_5 is important for carbohydrate processing as well as nervous system support.

Symptoms of vitamin B_5 deficiency include increased irritability, problems with sleep quality, weakness, and depression. It's unlikely that most people are significantly depleted of the vitamin due to diet, but many likely have suboptimal levels and show few or no symptoms.

Foods that can help raise B_5 levels include green vegetables (such as broccoli and asparagus) as well as yogurt and eggs.

Pyridoxine (vitamin B₆)

Vitamin B_6 (pyridoxine) is important for adrenal gland functioning; it's one of the B vitamins important in the production of adrenal hormones.

Low levels of vitamin B_6 can affect nerve function and are a risk factor for developing depression. Full deficiency of this vitamin is very rare in industrialized countries. A common symptom of B_6 deficiency is *peripheral neuropathy,* which causes numbness and tingling in the hands and feet. Note that certain medications can inhibit production of B_6; a common example is isoniazid (isonicotinylhydrazine, or INH), which is used in treating tuberculosis.

Foods with high vitamin B_6 content include fish, nuts, and seeds.

Cyanocobalamin (vitamin B₁₂)

Vitamin B_{12} (cyanocobalamin) is important for nerve function and cell health. Like all other B vitamins, vitamin B_{12} is important for the synthesis of adrenal hormones.

Causes of B_{12} deficiency include *pernicious anemia* (an autoimmune condition where the body forms antibodies against certain cells of the stomach responsible for the production and absorption of B_{12}) and certain medications; a common example is metformin (Glucophage), likely the most commonly prescribed medication for the treatment of diabetes.

Low levels of vitamin B_{12} are a risk factor for developing depression. Symptoms of B_{12} deficiency can include diarrhea, numbness and tingling in the hands and feet (neuropathy), dementia, and problems with balance and coordination. You can measure deficiency of this vitamin by obtaining a simple B_{12} level in the blood.

Foods high in B_{12} content include fish, poultry, and eggs.

Keeping an eye on vitamin C

Like vitamin B_5 in the preceding section, vitamin C is vital for adrenal gland function. Did you know that one of the highest concentrations of vitamin C in your body is in the adrenal glands? It's found in both in the adrenal cortex and in the adrenal medulla (see Chapter 2 for more about these areas). Vitamin C is necessary for the production of steroid hormones and the hormones of the adrenal medulla, including epinephrine and norepinephrine. A research article from the journal *Endocrine Research* in 2004 suggests that depletion of vitamin C can also affect the functioning of the mitochondria in the adrenal cortex.

Vitamin C is also important for bone health and the production of collagen (important for joint health) as well as for many cellular reactions. It's one of the best antioxidants to help protect the cell from damage from inflammation.

Scurvy is a condition caused by total body depletion of vitamin C. It's characterized by anemia, fatigue, and mouth ulcerations. Scurvy was more common in the distant past, but it's rare today.

One of the best food sources for vitamin C is fresh citrus fruits. Other foods include broccoli, cauliflower, kale, mustard greens, and Brussels sprouts.

Dealing with vitamin D

Vitamin D deficiency affects millions of people, both young and old. As you're likely aware, the primary sources of vitamin D are the sun and the diet. With advances in technology, many folks spend increasing amounts of time in front of the television, the computer, and other electronic devices. They don't play outside or participate in many outside activities, so they don't get much sun. Couple that with a diet of poor nutritional value, and it's no wonder that vitamin D levels are low.

The many important functions of vitamin D in the body include the following:

- ✔ **Bone health:** Vitamin D is essential in helping maintain the balance of calcium and phosphorous in your body. Low levels of vitamin D can contribute to osteoporosis.

  Vitamin D is likely very important in countering the effects of sustained cortisol secretion by the adrenal cortex. Remember that sustained cortisol production can cause weakening of the bone structure over time and increase the risk of developing osteoporosis.

- ✔ **Immune system regulation:** Low levels of vitamin D affect your immune system's ability to fight off infection. They're linked to ongoing inflammation and chronic illness.

- ✔ **Blood health:** Vitamin D deficiency has been linked to anemia.

- ✔ **Heart health:** Data suggests that low levels of vitamin D are a risk factor for heart disease.

- ✔ **Hormone production:** Lab studies suggest that low vitamin D levels may affect the ability of the adrenal medulla to produce its hormones, although this finding is somewhat controversial.

You can determine whether your vitamin levels are low by asking your healthcare provider to order a blood test. Given the most recent research in this area, most practitioners feel that vitamin D levels below 20 nanograms per milliliter (ng/mL) represent an absolute deficiency. In fact, most practitioners aim for a vitamin D level greater than 40 ng/mL.

Most people in the United States and other industrialized countries have low levels of vitamin D but don't show any symptoms. The key is that the levels aren't low enough to cause symptoms of deficiency, even though the levels aren't optimal. The goal is optimal health. Raising vitamin D levels mostly requires getting out in the sun on a daily basis and supplementing with vitamin D. See Chapter 11 for important points concerning supplementation of this important vitamin.

Obesity and nutritional deficiencies

You may associate nutritional deficiencies with people who look like just skin and bones, but nutrient deficiencies aren't experienced only by those who are severely underweight. People who are obese (with a body mass index over 30) or severely overweight can have deficiencies, too. Being "fat" doesn't mean being well-nourished.

In the United States, people are victims of overfeeding while undernourishing. They eat too much of the wrong things. The result is deficiencies in *micronutrients* (chemical elements necessary in small amounts), which are important in breaking the cycle of obesity. Micronutrients include some of the vitamins and minerals that we discuss in this chapter.

Evaluating vitamin E

Adrenal gland function is part of the hypothalamus, pituitary, and adrenal gland (HPA) axis (see Chapter 2 for details). Some lab-based studies suggest that vitamin E may be important in maximizing how these three organs communicate with one another. A study from the *Journal of Clinical Biochemistry and Nutrition* published in 2009 looked at rats that were vitamin E deficient. They found that the rats' adrenal glands didn't decrease cortisol secretion when they were supposed to, a hallmark of adrenal fatigue in humans. The conclusion drawn was that vitamin E was important in order for all the HPA organs to understand the signals they were sending and to react appropriately.

Vitamin E deficiency is rare in the United States, but with the poor diet, people likely need to supplement with vitamin E to support adrenal gland health. Foods high in vitamin E include green vegetables, nuts, and seeds.

Boning up on vitamin K

Vitamin K comes in two forms (K_1 and K_2) and has several important functions. A primary function is maintaining bone health. Vitamin K_2 is more specific to bone health; it helps inhibit the leaching of calcium from the bones and the resulting influx of calcium into the blood vessels. (Head to the earlier section "Looking at potassium and calcium" for details on calcium leaching.) I (coauthor Rich) think of vitamin K_2 as being part of my arsenal for maintaining the bones' health and integrity in adrenal fatigue because it helps protect against excess calcium loss.

Vitamin K_1 is related to blood vessel health. People who are taking the medicine warfarin (Coumadin), a blood thinner, may see lower levels of vitamin K_1.

The most common reasons for vitamin K deficiency are taking warfarin or having a malabsorption syndrome (such as celiac disease), which can affect the absorption of vitamin K in the small intestine. Low levels of vitamin K increase the risk of bleeding.

Foods high in vitamin K_2 include meat and poultry.

Part III
Treating Adrenal Fatigue

Five Alternative Therapies That Can Ease Adrenal Fatigue

- **Increase your vitamin C intake.** The adrenal glands have one of the highest concentrations of this vitamin in the human body, so they can't function optimally without it.

- **Take a vitamin B complex.** Many of the B vitamins, including vitamin B_5 (pantothenic acid), are essential for the production of adrenal hormones.

- **Boost your adrenal function with an adrenal adaptogen.** Herbs such as ashwagandha and eleuthero support adrenal gland health. You'll find yourself feeling great as well.

- **Provide the cells of your adrenal glands with an energy boost.** Supplements like pyrroloquinoline quinone (PQQ) and ubiquinone power up the cells' energy centers (mitochondria) to help keep your adrenal glands in peak condition.

- **Protect your bones.** Because sustained cortisol secretion is associated with bone thinning and osteoporosis, consider a good bone mineral supplement to keep your bones healthy and strong.

 Find out how you can reduce stress at work (and ease your adrenal fatigue) in a free article at www.dummies.com/extras/adrenalfatigue.

In this part...

- Find the best healthcare practitioner for you. Being diagnosed with adrenal fatigue requires working with a good healthcare practitioner, who should be willing to have an open and honest discussion with you about your symptoms. A qualified health-care practitioner may be a naturopathic physician, an integrative medicine physician, or a holistic health practitioner.

- Understand when you may need medication and hormone supplementation. For example, your blood pressure may be so low that you need meds to improve it.

- Look at alternative remedies, including minerals, vitamins, energy boosts to your cells, antioxidant support, and much more.

- Get the scoop on exercising right. You need to be careful when you start an exercise program. A regimen lower in intensity and shorter in duration can help you avoid muscle fatigue and decrease the risk of injury.

- See the secrets of managing stress in the workplace. Job-related stress is a significant component of adrenal fatigue; it makes you ill and can make you crazy. Employ strategies to reduce stress.

Chapter 9

Finding and Working with a Good Practitioner

In This Chapter

▶ Being an advocate for your health

▶ Knowing what to do if your doctor won't work with you

▶ Recognizing the holistic approach needed to treat adrenal fatigue

▶ Selecting a team of healthcare practitioners

▶ Making sure your team runs smoothly

*B*ecause adrenal fatigue is associated with so many other medical conditions (see Chapter 3 for details), it's important to find the right healthcare provider or team of practitioners. One of the biggest hurdles concerning the diagnosis and treatment of adrenal fatigue is finding a healthcare provider who's open and willing to work with you. You may find — or may have found already — that many physicians and other medical experts aren't aware of this condition or don't believe it exists.

In this chapter, you read about the healthcare providers you should seek out concerning the evaluation and treatment of adrenal fatigue. You also find out why a team approach may be just what the doctor ordered.

Taking an Active Role in Your Healthcare

Traditionally, patients simply did whatever their doctors advised. But the nature of the doctor-patient relationship has changed. The healthcare provider and patient now share in the decision-making process. For this relationship to work, your healthcare provider needs to listen to you and should be open to discussing new ideas concerning your health and wellness.

Even if your healthcare provider is unfamiliar with a particular healthcare concept, he or she should say something to the effect of "let me look this up and get back to you so we can talk about it."

When dealing with any healthcare provider, be sure to stick to your guns concerning your health. This is especially true if your provider doesn't believe your signs or symptoms. You know your body better than any practitioner; after all, you've been living in it all your life! The worst thing you can do, no matter what the condition, is to ignore your warning signs.

We would also caution you to avoid cutting healthcare providers out of the decision-making process. You want the decisions you make concerning your health to be informed ones. This means being aware of all your options. It also means you need to keep an open mind to the recommendations of your healthcare provider.

Many people search online for information concerning the signs and symptoms that they're experiencing. The Internet can be wealth of information; that being said, the *context* of the information in relation to your own personal health situation is important. Not all the signs and symptoms that you read about for a given diagnosis necessarily pertain to you.

The corollary to this is also true: Information that you read about online may provide just the right context for you to have an informed conversation with your doctor and/or other healthcare providers.

Taking Action If Your Doctor Won't Listen to You

Because the symptoms of adrenal fatigue can overlap other medical conditions, this syndrome can be difficult for many doctors to understand, let alone diagnose. Many physicians and healthcare providers aren't aware of this condition, and many don't believe that this condition truly exists.

Your doctor may tell you your symptoms are psychological. You may be told that your symptoms are so vague that they can't be linked to any medical condition. Guess what! Just because a clinician doesn't recognize the signs and symptoms of adrenal fatigue doesn't mean that the condition doesn't exist. For the longest time, many in the healthcare profession didn't believe that chronic pain syndromes, chronic fatigue syndrome, or fibromyalgia syndrome existed. Experts now know that these conditions are very real.

Why do many physicians not recognize adrenal fatigue? The model of training that most physicians undergo is a reductionist model. They begin by listing and organizing a person's presenting signs and symptoms. They then look for the one or two medical conditions that can fit those particular symptoms. If a particular set of symptoms doesn't fit the medical model, then the question of whether the presenting symptoms are even valid can arise. As the medical community learns more about genetics, nutrition, and the effects of stress and chronic inflammation, the way that doctors are practicing medicine is slowly being transformed.

The good news is that many changes are occurring in the education of doctors and other health professionals. There's now a focus on personalizing the interaction between doctor and patient. Healthcare practitioners are learning about the effects that nutrient deficiencies, environmental toxins, and stress have on people's adrenal and total body health. Individuals are different, and everyone can present differently.

The diagnosis of adrenal fatigue requires that a healthcare provider consider all diagnostic alternatives. It requires a holistic approach, which is why this diagnosis is often made by a holistic health practitioner or a physician trained in holistic health (see the next section for details on the holistic approach).

If you find that you're experiencing many of the conditions listed in this book but your doctor refuses to listen or is unwilling to work with you, you have two options: Either seek out another physician, or keep your physician but seek out the services of a holistic health practitioner to help you find out whether you have adrenal fatigue. In reality, people often have more than one healthcare provider.

Understanding the Holistic Approach to Treating Adrenal Fatigue

Adrenal fatigue can be diagnosed and treated only through a holistic approach. A holistic practitioner understands that body, mind, and spirit are interrelated and that all three need to be evaluated to achieve total wellness.

Any healthcare provider you deal with should use a holistic approach. This approach involves trying to restore balance to the body. If you have adrenal fatigue, multiple factors are likely causing your body to be out of balance. The goal is to first identify those causes. The next step is to formulate a treatment plan to correct them as best as possible. What does that approach involve?

✔ **Understanding the many testing modes:** Diagnosing adrenal fatigue is a comprehensive process, involving not only blood tests but also urine and salivary testing (see Chapter 5 for details). Interpreting these tests, especially the hormonal testing, often requires a certain level of expertise. Searching for causes of inflammation, testing for food sensitivities, and evaluating the acid-base balance and nutritional status are vital in the diagnosis and treatment of adrenal fatigue.

✔ **Treating beyond prescription medications:** Prescription medications do have their place in treating adrenal fatigue (see Chapter 10 for details); however, the treatment of adrenal fatigue is multifaceted, going beyond just writing a prescription. The healthcare provider you work with should have an understanding of nutrition and nutrition-based therapies. Your practitioner should work with you to develop a personalized approach. (Please refer to Chapter 11 to read about alternative remedies and treatments that can be used in the treatment of adrenal fatigue.)

✔ **Including exercise in the treatment plan:** Your healthcare provider should have an understanding of exercise and fitness. Creating an exercise plan of the right intensity and duration is crucial in treating adrenal fatigue. The wrong type of exercise program can actually worsen your symptoms! Please refer to Chapter 12 for information on developing a personalized exercise program.

✔ **Homing in on hormonal manipulation:** The practitioner that you work with should have some familiarity with hormones and hormonal treatments, because they're often part of the treatment plan for someone with adrenal fatigue (see Chapter 10 for details).

Choosing Experts for Your Team

Many patients with adrenal fatigue not only see more than one medical doctor but also see more than one holistic healthcare provider. The members of your healthcare team can include your medical doctor, your holistic practitioner, a nutritionist, and a practitioner dealing with the mind and the spirit. In this section, you read about some types of practitioners you may choose to work with.

One of the best ways to choose any healthcare practitioner is by word of mouth. Find out the experiences of other people who've worked with this particular practitioner. You can also check out websites, such as Angie's List, where people post their experiences with a particular healthcare practitioner.

A holistic practitioner

For holistic care, you can choose from so many holistic practitioners. Examples include naturopathic physicians, physicians certified in anti-aging medicine, integrative physicians, and homeopathic physicians. There's some degree of overlap among their roles; often the choice of holistic practitioner is based on patient preference, word-of-mouth referral, and/or prior patient or family experience with a certain type of holistic practitioner. You may choose to add more than one holistic practitioner to your team, based on your specific needs.

A naturopathic physician

A naturopathic physician is trained in *naturopathy,* a distinct field of medicine whose focus is on natural treatments, including the use of botanicals, homeopathic preparations, and nutrition to enable the body to heal itself. In some states, naturopathic physicians are licensed to prescribe medications; however, these physicians usually choose to prescribe natural remedies and lifestyle changes in most cases. The naturopathic physician's goal is to use approaches that support the natural healing of the body.

People often choose a naturopathic physician to provide a complementary approach to treating the conditions for which they also see their "regular doctor."

Naturopathic physicians undergo four years of premedical school training and then four years of post-graduate naturopathic medical school training. For example, the University of Bridgeport, Southwest College of Naturopathic Medicine, and Bastyr University offer four-year programs similar to medical school training. A graduate from this type of school has undergone rigorous classroom work in addition to bedside teaching and clinical rotations, just like doctors graduating from medical school.

For a listing of naturopathic physicians in your area, please visit www.naturopathic.org.

An anti-aging specialist

One of the most exciting new fields in medicine is *anti-aging.* The anti-aging specialist is trained in a holistic approach to body function, including hormone testing, which is one of the reasons that these specialists are excellent resources for people with adrenal fatigue. They've been specially trained to evaluate all aspects of adrenal function and to prescribe personalized treatment plans. Anti-aging experts seek to treat, prevent, and reverse medical conditions that shorten life span and to improve quality of life as people age.

Anti-aging specialists provide a comprehensive approach to care that can benefit everyone. That being said, because of their added expertise in adrenal function and hormone testing, women very much benefit from seeing this type of healthcare practitioner. Anti-aging specialists' expertise in bioidentical hormone replacement can dramatically improve the quality of life for many women.

A certified anti-aging specialist has completed a training program in anti-aging medicine. The University of South Florida has an excellent program. Note that many healthcare practitioners, including medical doctors (MDs), osteopathic physicians (DO), physician assistants (PA), nurse practitioners (NP), and PhDs, can undergo training in this field of medicine. You can find information on anti-aging training programs at www.a4m.com.

For help finding a practitioner certified in anti-aging medicine, visit www.worldhealth.net.

A practitioner of homeopathy

A practitioner of homeopathy doesn't prescribe drugs or surgery. *Homeopathy* is based on prescribing as little as possible to give the body just enough of what it needs to begin to heal. Homeopathy is similar to naturopathy in that practitioners of both forms of medicine believe that the body has an innate ability to heal itself. The homeopathic practitioner, however, often prescribes a natural substance in smaller amounts. Compared to the dosage of a natural supplement, homeopathic dosages are extremely minute. Homeopathic practitioners don't prescribe in terms of milligrams or grams; they prescribe in terms of dilutions (a dilution is likely exponentially smaller than a milligram).

I (coauthor Rich) have found homeopathy to be especially helpful for patients who don't tolerate medications. People who experience significant side effects to many medications and supplements, even in the smallest doses, often do well with homeopathy.

To find a practitioner of homeopathy, visit http://nationalcenterfor homeopathy.org/resources/practitioners.

A nutritionist

Nutrition is vital not only in the treatment of adrenal fatigue but also in total body health. Food is medicine; the right food has the power to heal. Treating adrenal fatigue effectively means improving your nutrition and eliminating the junk in your diet, in addition to lifestyle changes, supplements, medication, and/or hormonal replacement therapy.

Vitamin and nutritional deficiencies (see Chapter 8) are significant causes of adrenal fatigue. This condition won't get better without the right nutritional support.

If your healthcare provider isn't well-versed in nutrition (which is often the case), then we recommend a visit with a nutritionist. And in terms of general preventive health, we encourage routine visits to a nutritionist.

To find and choose a qualified nutritionist, try an online referral service, such as `www.eatright.org`. Another option is to contact your insurance company to see what nutrition services may be part of your plan. Many medical conditions, including diabetes, entitle you to a certain number of visits with a nutritionist.

A practitioner who deals with the mind and the spirit

Remember that the holistic approach involves more than just healing the body. Your mental, emotional, and spiritual states also need to be evaluated and treated. Renewal of the mind and spirit is crucial in the treatment of adrenal fatigue.

Yoga, meditation, and t'ai chi all are examples of therapies that strengthen the mind and the spirit. In addition, they're great ways to relieve the stress that leads to adrenal fatigue. You can find info on these meditative exercises in Chapter 12.

Yoga and t'ai chi instructors should be included as practitioners to help in the treatment of adrenal fatigue. Use resources such as `www.yogaalliance.org` and `www.patiencetaichi.com` to find out what types of instructors are available in your area. You should be able to find a school and instructor near you. Also ask your neighbors and friends for their recommendations.

Working Well with Your Team

If you're working with two or more practitioners, you're the MVP of your healthcare team. You should feel comfortable with the members of your team and be able to talk with them openly about any health concern that you have.

Maintaining communication

Many patients see their doctor and are reluctant to mention any supplements that they're taking or any other healthcare practitioners they're seeing. This truncated communication is a barrier to good, effective, comprehensive, and personalized care.

Because adrenal fatigue can be difficult to diagnose, it requires communication among all your providers. I (coauthor Rich) have called a patient's herbalist, homeopathic practitioner, and naturopathic physician, all in the name of continuity of care.

Never, ever, hesitate to tell your doctor anything. Fear of repercussions should not be a barrier to care. If you're seeing more than one healthcare provider, you need to maintain communication with all of them and facilitate communication among them. Withholding vital medical information can compromise your care.

Here are a couple of ways you can help promote communication among your healthcare providers:

✔ Keep copies of all your reports and lab tests from all your providers.

✔ Don't hesitate to ask a provider to call another provider on your team during an office visit to discuss aspects of your care. If you're seeing several providers in one day, sometimes they may not have the information concerning a change in the treatment plan from another provider.

Holding yourself accountable

Some patients abide by the old model, where they want to go the doctor to get fixed, like taking their car to a mechanic for a tune-up. Guess what! The treatment for adrenal fatigue involves more than being fixed. It requires you to make changes to improve your nutrition, reduce stress, and improve sleep as well as add supplements and make work and lifestyle changes. These changes help de-stress your adrenal glands and return you to total body balance.

All these changes require accountability on your part. After you and your healthcare team agree on a plan, you need to do your best to stick with it. This includes maintaining communication and keeping follow-up appointments. It means sticking with a nutrition and exercise program as best as you can and alerting your healthcare provider(s) of any problems that arise. You want to be proactive in your healthcare, not just reactive. Only by doing so can you be successful in overcoming adrenal fatigue.

Chapter 10

Using Medications and Hormone Supplementation

In This Chapter

▶ Helping low blood pressure

▶ Reviewing bioidentical hormone replacement

*T*he treatment for adrenal fatigue is multifaceted. It can involve a combination of medications and hormone replacement as well as changes in nutrition and vitamin/mineral supplements (see Chapter 11). In this chapter, you see the role of medications and hormone replacement in treating adrenal fatigue. You find out about raising low blood pressure — the use of prescription medications and hormonal supplements to help keep your blood pressure normal. In addition, you get a detailed picture of hormone replacement, including a discussion of *bioidentical* hormone replacement therapy.

The medications and hormones that we discuss in this chapter have several purposes. They're used to treat symptoms of adrenal fatigue as well as to supplement the hormones that the adrenal glands are unable to produce in sufficient amounts because of adrenal fatigue.

Understand that everyone's adrenal needs are different; some people may need to be on medications and hormone supplementation longer than others. People on bioidentical hormone replacement, especially those who are older, may need to be on these supplements for a long time if not for life.

Raising Low Blood Pressure with Medications and Steroid Hormones

In the advanced stages of adrenal fatigue, low blood pressure is common. You may need a prescription medication to increase your blood pressure, or you may need to supplement with an adrenal steroid hormone. In cases of adrenal exhaustion, you may need both types of supplementation to help keep your blood pressure in a normal range.

One way to see whether you're responding to any of the meds in this section is to check your blood pressure while you're lying, sitting, and standing. Sometimes when you stand up, you may have an abrupt decrease in blood pressure. As you read in Chapter 4, dizziness and lightheadedness commonly occur in adrenal fatigue. If your medications are working, you shouldn't experience dizziness and lightheadedness when standing up and you shouldn't see a difference in the blood pressure readings taken in different positions (sitting, standing). If you do, you need to talk with your healthcare practitioner about modifying your medication dosage.

In some people, the blood pressure meds can raise blood pressure even at low doses; this occurs in patients who still have some degree of adrenal reserve. You should monitor your blood pressure on a regular basis with a blood pressure cuff and call your healthcare provider if you notice your blood pressure numbers increasing beyond a normal range. Your medication and/or supplement program may need to be adjusted.

Minding midodrine

Midodrine (ProAmitine) is a prescription medication taken orally. It works on the blood vessels to help normalize blood pressure. How does it work? It stimulates *alpha receptors* on your blood vessels, causing the arteries to narrow. This narrowing, called *vasoconstriction,* helps increase your blood pressure.

Because midodrine is a short-acting medication, you typically take it several times a day. Common times are 8:00 a.m., 1:00 p.m., and 6:00 p.m. Because everyone responds differently to this medication, it's often prescribed first at a low dose (normally 2.5 milligrams two to three times a day) and increased slowly. The maximum dose is 10 milligrams three times a day.

Avoid taking midodrine late at night before you go to bed. In some people, it can cause *supine hypertension,* in which your blood pressure increases quickly when you're lying flat. If you're taking midodrine, lie down with the head of your bed elevated at 30 degrees to avoid supine hypertension. Midodrine can dramatically increase the risk of developing very high blood pressure while you're sleeping, so many healthcare practitioners prescribe that midodrine be taken no later than 6 p.m.

Supplementing with salt tablets

Salt craving is a symptom of adrenal fatigue (see Chapter 4 for details). Sometimes the salt craving can be so bad and the blood pressure so low that supplementing with salt is necessary. Salt raises blood pressure and blood volume.

One option for replacing the body's salt deficit is through salt tablets. I (coauthor Rich) usually prescribe tablets of sodium chloride (yes, table salt) when the blood pressure is very low and the person isn't able or likely to increase salt intake on his or her own.

The most common prescribed starting dosage of sodium chloride is 1 gram a day. A person may eventually be prescribed 2 or 3 grams of salt a day, often to be taken in divided doses during the day (usually half in the morning and half in the evening).

If you're on salt tablets, monitor your blood pressure on a daily basis. If you notice higher than normal blood pressure readings, contact your healthcare practitioner to see whether the dose needs to be adjusted.

Handling hydrocortisone

If hormonal testing reveals that your adrenal glands can no longer produce adequate amounts of cortisol (a hormone we discuss in Chapter 2), you may need to supplement with hydrocortisone. Hydrocortisone is a *steroid hormone,* normally produced by the *zona fasciculata* of the adrenal cortex. If your adrenals are exhausted, you probably aren't producing enough cortisol, so you're probably going to benefit from supplementation. One of the benefits of hydrocortisone is that it can normalize blood pressure as well.

Your options are a prescription medication or an adrenal-based steroid. Hydrocortisone is the most common prescription steroid hormone replacement prescribed. It's taken orally, usually twice a day.

Your healthcare provider determines the hydrocortisone dosing based on your stage of adrenal fatigue, blood pressure, and other symptoms. For example, late stages of adrenal fatigue often require higher doses (and earlier stages, lower doses). A typical, everyday dosing regimen is 5 milligrams in the morning and 2.5 milligrams at night. Your dosing schedule may be different, of course, depending on your individual needs.

If you've been prescribed hydrocortisone, talk with your doctor to find out whether your dose needs to increase in times of severe stress, such as when you're admitted to the hospital for a really bad infection. Ask whether you need to have the hydrocortisone given intravenously (via the vein) when you're in the hospital. The intravenous hydrocortisone can help you avoid going into adrenal shock while you're being treated for the underlying infection.

Using fludrocortisone

Fludrocortisone (Florinef) is a commonly prescribed steroid hormone. Think of fludrocortisone as working like a synthetic aldosterone (see Chapter 2 for details on aldosterone). It primarily raises blood pressure by increasing the body's absorption of sodium.

This medication is taken orally. Most healthcare practitioners start with a low dose of 0.1 milligrams per day. This can be increased to be taken twice a day at the same dose.

If tests show that your aldosterone levels (in addition to your cortisol levels) are low, your healthcare practitioner may talk to you about taking an aldosterone substitute like fludrocortisone. It will help raise your blood pressure, but the picture isn't entirely rosy — this medication can have significant side effects that you need to be aware of:

- **Really high blood pressure:** If your blood pressure readings are higher than normal, you may need to talk with your healthcare practitioner about adjusting the dose. You need to monitor your blood pressure on a daily basis.

- **Increased swelling in the legs (edema):** If you have a history of congestive heart failure (CHF), this medication may not be a great option, because it can cause salt and water retention. That's bad. The retention of salt and water is the cause of edema.

- **Weight gain:** If you're on fludrocortisone, weigh yourself daily. If you see rapid weight gain — more than 2 pounds in two consecutive days — talk with your healthcare provider about adjusting your dose. Weight gain that occurs quickly is often fluid weight (likely the byproduct of salt and water retention).

Using compounding pharmacies

Many naturally based healthcare practitioners use and recommend compounding pharmacies. A *compounding pharmacy* literally makes medications (that is, it *compounds* them). The compounding pharmacist can create a medication from scratch, especially if the dose of the med or supplement needs to be personalized, which is often the case with hormonal therapies.

To find a compounding pharmacy near you, check out www.ecompoundingpharmacy.com. Many pharmacies have mail-order service; contact a compounding pharmacy in your area to see whether it offers this service.

The weight gain associated with this medication can increase the risk of developing fluid overload; an example is *congestive heart failure (CHF)*, which is a buildup of fluid in the lungs.

✔ **Low potassium (hypokalemia):** Fludrocortisone can cause urinary excretion of potassium (like high levels of aldosterone would), leading to low potassium levels in the body. If you're taking this medication, your potassium levels likely need to be checked routinely, and you may be asked to supplement with potassium as well.

In addition to fludrocortisone, a natural form of aldosterone is available. It can be difficult to get in the United States, although you may find it in compounding pharmacies (see the sidebar "Using compound pharmacies"). This form of aldosterone is considered natural because it's identical to the human form of aldosterone and is derived from plant sources.

Hearing loss, which may be associated with low levels of aldosterone, can be treated with aldosterone replacement. Just as mineralocorticoid receptors are in the adrenal glands, the same receptors are in the ear. Isn't it amazing how everything in the body is interrelated?

Replacing Sex Hormones

Hormone testing (see Chapter 5) can show whether you need hormone replacement. In this section, you read about *general* guidelines concerning hormone replacement; we explain the basics of bioidentical hormone replacement therapy and list some hormones (specifically, sex hormones) that can be replaced.

Because of the complex nature of adrenal gland physiology, too low or too high of a dose of hormones can be counterproductive. Here are a few facets of hormone replacement that you need to be aware of:

✔ Everyone's hormonal needs are different, so the treatment needs to be personalized.

✔ When you begin hormone treatment, your healthcare practitioner will likely follow your hormone levels to see whether your dosing needs to be adjusted periodically.

✔ Increasing the dose of one hormone can alter the levels of other hormones. For example, DHEA supplementation can change the levels of testosterone and/or estradiol in some people. Everything can affect everything else, so be aware of possible side effects with hormone supplementation.

✔ Even though your hormonal profile may suggest that hormone replacement is necessary, your personal health situation may prevent the use of hormone replacement. For example, prostate cancer precludes testosterone replacement in men.

Do not take random doses of hormones yourself. Hormone replacement should be done under the guidance of a qualified health professional. See Chapter 9 for information on seeking out a qualified provider.

Before you begin: Understanding bioidentical hormone replacement therapy

If tests indicate that you require hormone replacement, your healthcare practitioner will likely discuss prescribing bioidentical hormones. This treatment is called *bioidentical hormone replacement therapy,* or BHRT. *Bioidentical hormones,* which are derived from plant sources, are molecularly and chemically identical to the hormones your body makes. Because bioidentical hormones are identical to your body's hormones, they're thought to be safer than synthetic hormones, which tend to have a worse side-effect profile.

If you've been prescribed bioidentical hormones, you need to obtain them at a specialized pharmacy called a *compounding pharmacy*. There, the pharmacists are experts in preparing natural products. (See the earlier sidebar "Using compounding pharmacies" for details.)

Bioidentical hormones can be dosed in different ways. Many practitioners prefer the topical forms (such as a patch or cream) to the oral form, despite the convenience of the oral form. Here's how the forms compare:

✔ **Oral formulation:** All bioidentical hormones are available in oral form; however, many healthcare practitioners don't recommend oral dosing to their patients as first-line treatment, because a portion of such meds is broken down by stomach acid and the major part is metabolized by the liver. As a result, a patient is likely to absorb only 30 percent of the medication.

Hormone binding also plays a big role in hormone levels. When a protein in the blood binds to a hormone, the hormone level in the blood decreases, decreasing the hormone's efficacy. For example, when you take an oral dose of estrogen, your body may produce more of the protein *sex hormone binding globulin (SHBG),* which may alter the levels of other sex hormones. That's why being under the care of a qualified practitioner and having your hormone levels followed is so important.

✔ **Transdermal patch:** A patch produces a slow and continuous release of a hormone, bypassing the liver's processing. With the patch form, the levels of SHBG don't increase as much, making the treatment less likely to interfere with the levels of other hormones.

One disadvantage of a transdermal patch is that local skin irritation may occur. Often, you need to rotate the patch site with each application.

✔ **Creams:** A cream is a very common form of hormonal preparation. Note that with estrogen (estradiol) and progesterone, vaginal creams are preferred. The vaginal mucosa (the mucus membrane) is a highly vascular area, and the hormone is able to reach effective levels in the bloodstream rather quickly. Many healthcare providers prefer creams.

A preparation may contain a combination of hormones — progesterone and estrogen, for example. A combination preparation (such as a combination transdermal patch) is convenient, but it can be troublesome if your provider needs to make adjustments to one part of the preparation. So despite the convenience, separate hormones are usually prescribed separately.

Pursuing pregnenolone

Pregnenolone is called a precursor hormone. It helps make other adrenal hormones (such as DHEA and testosterone, which we discuss later in this chapter), and it also acts on its own.

If your pregnenolone levels are low, your healthcare provider may talk to you about supplementing. Most healthcare practitioners prefer an oral form of this hormone, which is taken daily. The benefits of taking pregnenolone can include the following:

✔ Improvement in cognition and memory

✔ Increase in energy and overall improved sense of well-being

✔ Improvement in sleep quality

The potential side effects of taking pregnenolone are related to the hormones your body may convert it into. Possible side effects include the following:

- **Arrhythmia (palpitations or abnormal heart rhythms):** In some people, pregnenolone supplementation may cause an irregular heartbeat. This may be related to the fact that the body can change pregnenolone into DHEA, which at high doses may increase the risk of developing an abnormal heart rhythm. (See the next section for info on DHEA.)
- **Insomnia:** In some people, pregnenolone may cause insomnia, especially at higher doses. Insomnia is thought to be related to the pregnenolone itself.
- **Headaches:** Some people complain of headaches when taking this medication over a long period of time or when starting at higher doses.

Getting the pregnenolone dose right is very important, because low doses decrease the risk of side effects. A typical starting dose of pregnenolone is 5 to 10 milligrams once a day. The dosage is slowly increased, based on your hormone levels.

Dealing with DHEA

Many personalized hormonal treatment plans involve a prescription for dehydroepiandrosterone (DHEA) because levels of this hormone may be low in someone with adrenal fatigue. Your body converts DHEA to testosterone and estradiol, both of which we discuss later in this chapter.

The benefits of DHEA supplementation can include the following:

- Improved sleep quality
- Possible help in treating depression

DHEA is prescribed most commonly in an oral form. Starting doses are approximately 5 milligrams once a day, usually taken in the morning.

If you're prescribed DHEA, you can increase the absorption by taking it with an oil (olive oil or the omega oils, for example). Do not increase the absorption without first speaking with your healthcare provider.

Now, about those side effects. . . . Be aware of the potential risks of taking DHEA:

✔ **Abnormal heart rhythms:** Abnormal heart rhythms may happen, especially at higher doses.

✔ **Increased blood pressure and elevated cholesterol levels:** Be sure to monitor your blood pressure and follow your cholesterol levels.

✔ **Insomnia:** In some people, DHEA supplementation can worsen sleep problems, including insomnia.

✔ **Facial hair:** DHEA can increase the levels of estradiol and/or testosterone. If you're a woman and you find yourself growing facial hair while taking DHEA, you may need to stop using the supplement and obtain a repeat DHEA-S level; your practitioner will likely need to adjust your dosage.

✔ **Hair loss:** Excessive use of DHEA can cause hair loss. Given that the hormone may cause the growth of facial hair, this is hardly fair, but it's the truth.

The treatment of adrenal fatigue isn't about hormonal supplementation alone; it's the *incorporation* of hormonal supplementation into a complete adrenal recovery program. Here are some natural ways to improve DHEA levels:

✔ Reducing stress can increase hormone levels. Chapter 6 has pointers on reducing stress in your daily life.

✔ Exercise — along with a diet that's mostly plants, low in carbohydrates, low in omega-6 fatty acids, and high in omega-3 fish oils — can also increase DHEA levels.

Teasing out testosterone

If your testosterone levels are low, your healthcare practitioner will probably suggest testosterone replacement. The benefits of testosterone therapy (usually in men) include the following:

✔ Improved energy levels

✔ Increased libido

✔ Improved mood and sense of well-being

(Note that testosterone can be prescribed for a woman, depending on her hormonal profile.)

The most common type of testosterone replacement is either a gel form or a patch. Your practitioner will follow your levels after you start on testosterone therapy. One example of a gel form, Androderm, is often applied to the skin on a daily basis. Modifications in dosing depend on follow-up testing of testosterone and other hormonal levels. If your testosterone level is still low, for example, the gel form can be applied to the skin twice a day.

Here are some potential side effects of testosterone therapy:

- ✔ It can affect sleep quality. It may worsen symptoms of sleep apnea in some people, particularly if they haven't been treated for this condition.
- ✔ It may increase the risk of heart disease.
- ✔ It may increase the risk of developing certain types of skin problems, such as pimples and acne.
- ✔ In some men, the liver may process (or metabolize) the testosterone into estrogen. This can cause men to develop breasts and gain weight. That's why following the hormonal profile after testosterone replacement begins is so important.

If you have a history of cancer, especially prostate cancer, then testosterone replacement may not be for you. Testosterone can increase the growth of prostate tissue, which is the last thing you want if you have prostate cancer.

Adding estrogen

If your estrogen levels are low, supplementation may be a good idea. One of the most common forms of natural supplementation comes in the form of *estradiol,* which is made from soy. Benefits may include the following:

- ✔ Helping to maintain and/or improve bone density (that is, decreasing the risk of developing osteoporosis)
- ✔ Heart protection
- ✔ Improved memory and cognition

There are many ways to administer *estradiol.* Two of the most common ways are the transdermal patch and cream. Estradiol cream doesn't dramatically increase the risk of cancer the way the oral form of estrogen may do. Another way to administer estradiol is a gel form that's given once daily; hormone levels are followed, and the dose of the gel can be adjusted as needed.

One of the main reservations about prescribing estrogen in the past came from the increased risk of breast and endometrial cancer. This concern came about from the Nurses' Health Study, which has followed 230,000 female registered nurses since 1976 to assess risk factors for cancer and cardiovascular disease. The first study surveyed 122,000 women over the course of about

10 years. It demonstrated that the use of estrogen in addition to the use of synthetic progesterone increased the risk of developing breast cancer. The results of the study also concluded that estrogen given alone increased the risk of cancer.

A study from *Postgraduate Medicine* in 2009 did a review of the available papers concerning the safety of bioidentical hormone supplementation, namely estradiol and progesterone (discussed in the next section). The authors concluded that the use of *bioidentical* hormones was associated with a decreased risk of breast cancer and heart disease compared to the synthetic and animal-derived forms of the hormones.

Probing progesterone

Progesterone is a hormone important for regulating the menstrual cycle, maintaining mood and thinking, and regulating sleep in women. The benefits of progesterone therapy include the following:

- ✔ Improved sleep quality
- ✔ Improved memory and cognition, including resolution of brain fog
- ✔ Improved mood

There are many ways to prescribe progesterone, including orally and in the form of a cream. Most healthcare practitioners prefer progesterone cream because it seems to have fewer side effects. The cream is often applied on a daily basis.

The side effects of using progesterone can include the following:

- ✔ **Sleeping too much:** Progesterone deficiency is associated with insomnia. Too much progesterone can cause the opposite problem: increased drowsiness and lethargy. If you have this symptom, you may need to have your dosage adjusted.

- ✔ **Gaining weight:** This side effect isn't felt to be a major issue, because the weight gains aren't huge.

Certain vitamin and mineral deficiencies can decrease your body's ability to produce progesterone naturally. The good news is that B vitamins (especially vitamin B_6) and vitamin C can help boost your adrenal production of progesterone. In addition, zinc is important in treating progesterone deficiency, so supplementing with zinc can also help boost your body's progesterone levels. Foods high in magnesium can increase progesterone levels, too. (Flip to Chapter 11 for more on using vitamins to treat adrenal fatigue.)

Foods and herbs that increase the estrogen levels in the body may also have an effect of *lowering* progesterone levels. Avoid certain herbal supplements, including black cohosh, licorice, saw palmetto, and hops.

Chapter 11

Assessing Natural Treatments

- -

In This Chapter

▶ Dealing with mineral and vitamin depletion

▶ Energizing your cells

▶ Decreasing inflammation and putting your pH into balance

▶ Handling intestinal health and sleeping well

▶ Using herbs and considering detox

- -

*Y*ou can combat adrenal fatigue in many ways, including correcting mineral and vitamin deficiencies and normalizing intestinal flora. You can reduce inflammation, give your body antioxidant support, and alkalinize your pH. Of course, directly supporting the adrenal glands is always valuable, too.

This chapter gives you information on natural treatments for adrenal fatigue. You may call these remedies *alternative medicine,* but they're rapidly becoming the mainstream approach to making and keeping you well.

Please be aware that your treatment for adrenal fatigue should be personalized. You may need just one or two of the treatments in this chapter, or you may need a good number of them. Work with your healthcare practitioner to find a treatment plan that's right for you, and consider having a compounding pharmacy create your supplements to decrease the number of pills you take. To find a compounding pharmacy, visit www.ecompoundingpharmacy.com.

Your degree of adrenal fatigue and how you respond to the treatment will determine whether you need long-term supplementation. Continued vitamin and nutritional support is often recommended.

Managing Mineral Depletion

If you have adrenal fatigue, you're likely deficient in one or more minerals essential for health. Chronic inflammation, diet, and intestinal dysbiosis are common reasons for mineral depletion in adrenal fatigue.

To overcome a mineral deficiency, the first step is to change your diet. If dietary changes aren't enough, then supplementing is reasonable. However, you won't get the full benefit of nutrient supplementation unless you change your diet, because supplements alone can't treat adrenal fatigue. Dietary changes are crucial in restoring total-body health and the health of your adrenal glands. (Flip to Chapter 8 for details on minerals' roles in adrenal fatigue.)

The key minerals are magnesium, potassium, and calcium. Trace minerals include zinc, chromium, and selenium. Note that many, if not all, of the mineral supplements are available over-the-counter. Please consult your healthcare provider before starting any regimen.

Replacing magnesium

In general, healthcare practitioners recommended that you take in at least 600 to 800 milligrams of magnesium a day. Great dietary sources of magnesium include leafy green vegetables, seeds (sunflower and sesame, for example), and nuts (such as almonds and Brazil nuts).

If you're told that your magnesium levels are low after testing (a normal range is 1.6 to 2.6 milligrams per deciliter [mg/dL]), then you likely need to supplement. The goal of many healthcare practitioners is to have your magnesium level be at least 2.1 to 2.2 mg/dL to ensure optimal magnesium levels in the body. Many people need to take a magnesium supplement to get their levels higher.

Be aware that not all magnesium is created the same. The body absorbs different types of magnesium at different rates. For example, the body absorbs only a small amount of the magnesium in magnesium oxide, a commonly prescribed formulation.

Ask your healthcare provider to prescribe a supplement that's highly absorbed by the body, such as the following:

- **Chelated magnesium:** Chelated magnesium is a form of magnesium without the heavy metals. Normal starting doses are 200 milligrams twice a day. Coauthor Rich likes to use this form, which is well-tolerated. As with many forms of magnesium, diarrhea and loose stools are possible side effects.

✔ **Magnesium malate:** This combination of magnesium and malic acid is a well-tolerated form of magnesium that provides energy to the cells. As you may recall from your biology class in high school, the *mitochondria* are the powerhouses of the cell. Both magnesium and malic acid provide the energy necessary to make the mitochondria work optimally in the cell. This dynamic combination of magnesium and malic acid is highly recommended to anyone with adrenal fatigue.

More than 50 percent of people with fibromyalgia have associated adrenal fatigue, and I (coauthor Rich) think that anyone with fibromyalgia should strongly consider magnesium malate. In one study from the *Journal of Rheumatology* published in 1995, a combination of magnesium and malic acid not only reduced pain and tenderness in people with fibromyalgia but also improved their ability to function on a daily basis.

Magnesium malate comes in many forms. I prefer a dose of approximately 200 milligrams taken in divided doses throughout the day; this helps to enhance absorption. Magnesium malate can be taken with food.

Be aware that for some people, taking magnesium orally causes intestinal upset, including diarrhea. If you develop diarrhea soon after you start taking a magnesium supplement, inform your healthcare practitioner as soon as possible.

Magnesium is well-absorbed through the skin, so it can be administered topically as a gel or oil that's rubbed on the arms or legs on a daily basis. For people who have severe magnesium deficiency, I usually prescribe both an oral formulation and a topical gel. Some people experience a rash with magnesium oil, but the rash seems to be less common with the gel. For people who don't tolerate any form of oral magnesium, I recommend applying the gel twice a day.

In a few people, magnesium levels remain low despite the oral and topical (skin) forms of supplementation. In those cases, when the magnesium depletion is severe, I've had to prescribe magnesium to be given intravenously. This usually requires that the patient go to the short procedure unit of the hospital. The dose is usually 2 to 4 grams of magnesium sulfate over a few hours.

Knowing your potassium

Most adults don't consume enough potassium in their diets. Many healthcare practitioners recommend that the average adult consume approximately 4,000 to 4,500 milligrams of potassium a day. If you have certain medical conditions, such as kidney disease, the amount of potassium that you consume will likely need to be less. Speak with your healthcare practitioner concerning the amount of potassium you should be consuming on a daily basis.

Leafy green vegetables are excellent sources of potassium. However, after testing, your healthcare practitioner may tell you that you need a prescription potassium supplement. A prescribed form I like is potassium chloride. Because it comes in capsule form (as opposed to tablets, which tend to be large), it's easy to swallow, and it's usually well-tolerated.

Another option for potassium replacement is potassium iodide. Many people are deficient in iodine, which they need for adequate thyroid function, so the combination of potassium and iodine is useful. Speak with your healthcare provider to see whether this form of potassium replacement may be the right one for you.

Oral potassium supplements usually come in pill or capsule form. One common prescription form is potassium chloride. Potassium is measured in the blood in units of milliequivalents per liter (mEq/L); common prescription doses are usually 10 to 20 mEq taken twice daily. This dose may need to be modified, depending on your potassium needs. Your healthcare practitioner will order blood work to follow your potassium levels and make adjustments to how much potassium you need to take.

Choosing your calcium wisely

In the setting of adrenal fatigue, getting adequate calcium is necessary to help offset the negative effects of sustained cortisol production on your bone health. In general, most adults require about 1,000 milligrams of calcium a day. If you're over the age of 50, the daily calcium requirement increases to 1,200 milligrams a day.

Choose your calcium wisely. Your best bet is to increase the amount of leafy green vegetables in your diet, because they're generally good sources of calcium. Seeds and nuts also have excellent calcium content. Many of the same foods are also an excellent source of magnesium.

Yogurt can be an excellent source of calcium as well. A study from the journal *Nutrition Research* in 2013 reviewed the many beneficial health properties of yogurt. The authors concluded that people who consumed yogurt on a daily basis had better levels of calcium, potassium, and trace nutrients compared to those who did not. They also noted that regular yogurt intake helps to improve blood pressure, lower blood glucose levels, and lower cholesterol and triglyceride levels.

I (coauthor Rich) recommend that you minimize obtaining your calcium from a dairy-derived calcium supplement, pending further study in this area. A few studies have suggested that taking calcium in this form may increase the risk of developing heart disease as well as increasing the risk of developing calcium in the blood vessels (also known as *vascular calcification*). If your healthcare practitioner advises that you take calcium supplements, know that several nutraceutical companies have developed vegetarian forms of calcium; vegetarian sources may be better absorbed and handled by the body. Some even combine calcium, magnesium, and other trace minerals and vitamins, including vitamins C, D, and K_2.

Many supplements combine calcium and magnesium (see the earlier section "Replacing magnesium"). One big advantage of this combination is that it minimizes the potential side effects of both supplements. Calcium is known to cause constipation, and magnesium is known to cause diarrhea. If you take calcium and magnesium together, the gastrointestinal effects tend to cancel each other out.

If you need to supplement your calcium intake, I'd recommend looking for a vegetarian calcium formulation. Many formulations contain calcium doses that sum to 800 milligrams. For example, in one common vegetarian formulation of calcium, four capsules is the equivalent of 800 milligrams of calcium; I recommend taking two capsules twice a day. Again, speak with your healthcare provider. Depending on your dietary intake of calcium, the amount of calcium supplementation you require may be more or less.

Zeroing in on zinc and other trace minerals

Three trace minerals (zinc, chromium, and selenium) sometimes need replacement if testing shows you have low levels. When supplementing with micronutrients (in this case, microminerals), correct dosing is very important. With micronutrients, too little of a nutrient can be just as bad as too much of one. For example, low zinc levels can cause diarrhea, decrease your appetite, and impair your immune system. Taking too much zinc can cause similar symptoms, including nausea and diarrhea.

Zinc

Major zinc deficiencies are associated with at least 8 chronic diseases, and minor deficiencies are associated with at least 11 conditions. One of the best forms of zinc supplement is a chelated colloidal form, because it tends to be better absorbed. It's taken orally once a day.

Know that taking too much zinc can affect your body's ability to absorb copper (but don't stress about it, because stress contributes to adrenal fatigue). Also be aware that taking prescription medications, such as the following, may affect the ability of your intestine to absorb zinc:

✔ Doxycycline, a commonly prescribed antibiotic

✔ Fluoroquinolones, including levofloxacin and ciprofloxacin

Chromium

Insufficient dietary intake of chromium may impair glucose tolerance. The supplement chromium picolinate can help normalize blood sugars in the setting of adrenal fatigue. If you're finding that your blood glucose levels are higher than normal (which can occur in the early phases of adrenal fatigue) or are experiencing problems with hypoglycemia (which can occur in the later stages of adrenal fatigue), consider speaking with your healthcare provider about adding chromium to your treatment regimen. I (coauthor Rich) strongly encourage people with diabetes to use this supplement, too.

This supplement is usually taken once a day. I tend to begin with a lower dose (100 to 200 micrograms) of chromium daily and slowly increase to a maximum dose of 400 micrograms. For someone in the early phase of adrenal fatigue, I may start at the lower dose of 100 micrograms daily and follow blood glucose levels closely. Should you have diabetes, you need to watch your blood sugar levels carefully whenever you add a new therapy or change dosage.

Selenium

Selenium is important for many processes in the cell, especially for maintaining thyroid function. In general, selenium supplementation shouldn't exceed 200 micrograms a day. Too much selenium can cause nausea, diarrhea, and hair loss, among other conditions. It can be taken once daily, usually in capsule form.

Taking Your Vitamins

The best source of vitamins is food. Fruits and vegetables provide excellent antioxidant support in addition to supplying vitamins and other nutrients. For example, broccoli contains *sulforaphane,* a potent antioxidant that has anticancer and anti-infection properties.

However, if you have adrenal fatigue, then you need to consider vitamin supplementation. Most people with adrenal fatigue are likely depleted of important vitamins and minerals. Supplementing with the vitamins in this section — the B vitamins and vitamins C, D, E, and K — can help you restore your adrenal glands to health. (Check out Chapter 8 for info on the following vitamins' roles in adrenal fatigue and some tips for increasing your vitamin intake with food.)

Not all vitamins are created equal. The quality of the vitamins you take makes all the difference in how well they work in your body. Here are three characteristics of synthetic versus natural vitamins you should be aware of:

- **Ingredients:** Pay attention to the ingredients in vitamin supplements. Many synthetic vitamins may have other chemicals (used in the process of making them) that you don't want in your body. You can obtain most natural vitamins you need from a reputable health food store. Again, it's important to speak with your healthcare provider concerning the right type of vitamins for you.

- **Digestion:** Compared to natural vitamins, synthetic vitamins are harder for the stomach and intestine to break down.

- **Absorption:** Synthetic vitamins are chemically made and are often not as well absorbed as natural vitamins. A lot has to do with the preparation of the vitamin itself. Because the compounds in a natural vitamin are very similar to those found in food, they're easier to digest and absorb.

The vitamins in this section are taken orally unless otherwise specified.

Developing a B complex

Many diets are devoid of B vitamins. Because of the importance of the B vitamins for adrenal health, I (coauthor Rich) think everyone should take a B-complex supplement.

A good vitamin B complex has all the essential B vitamins your adrenal glands require, including thiamine (B_1), riboflavin (B_2), niacin (B_3), pantothenic acid (B_5), pyridoxine (B_6), and cyanocobalamin (B_{12}). The good news is that a high-quality vitamin B complex aids in the prevention of adrenal fatigue.

If you're experiencing any of the symptoms of adrenal fatigue (see Chapter 4), then you'll likely need to supplement some of these B vitamins at a higher dose:

- **Thiamine (B_1):** Start at a dose of 25 milligrams once a day.

- **Riboflavin (B_2):** Start at a dose of 200 milligrams once a day.

- **Niacin (B_3):** Start at a dose of 25 milligrams once a day.

- **Pantothenic acid (B_5):** Start at a dose of 500 to 1,000 milligrams a day; this can be taken twice a day in divided doses.

- **Pyridoxine (B_6):** Start at a dose of 50 milligrams once a day.

- **Cyanocobalamin (B_{12}):** This can be taken by mouth or under the tongue (*sublingually*). A good starting amount is 250 micrograms once a day for both the oral and sublingual formulations.

Seeing vitamin C

Vitamin C is super important for adrenal gland function. If your diet is low in vitamin C, then you may need to supplement in order to obtain the optimal amount to prevent adrenal fatigue. I (coauthor Rich) recommend taking vitamin C at a dose of 1,000 to 2,000 milligrams a day to provide the nutrient support that the adrenal glands need to deal with daily stresses.

If you have symptoms of adrenal fatigue, then you may need more vitamin C to nourish the adrenal glands — your dose may be as high as 4,000 to 5,000 milligrams a day. Ask your healthcare professional. You can take this vitamin twice a day in divided doses.

If you have kidney disease or are on dialysis, take a smaller dose of vitamin C. For someone with kidney disease, the normal dose is on the order of 250 to 500 milligrams a day. For symptoms of adrenal fatigue in this specific patient population, I recommend starting at 1,000 milligrams a day and *slowly* increasing.

Normalizing vitamin D levels

Vitamin D deficiency is at epidemic levels in the United States as well as in other industrialized nations, so vitamin D supplementation is usually a good idea. The goal of vitamin D therapy is to get your vitamin D level to greater than 40 nanograms per milliliter (ng/mL). Some experts recommend aiming for 50 ng/mL.

How much vitamin D do you need to take on a daily basis? The answer to that question is *enough*. That is, you need enough vitamin D to get your vitamin D levels above 40 ng/mL. Here are some basics about vitamin D supplementation:

- There are two forms of vitamin D replacement: vitamin D_2 and vitamin D_3. The former is derived from animals, and the latter is derived from plants. There's nothing wrong with either form, but I (coauthor Rich) tend to use vitamin D_3.

What about the sun? Excellent question! The sun is a great source of vitamin D. All you need is 15 minutes of sun exposure daily to get mega doses of vitamin D. Fifteen minutes of sun can give you 20,000 units of vitamin D. The key is to avoid getting sunburn.

✔ A maintenance dose of vitamin D_3 that everyone should be taking (with a few exceptions) is 1,000 to 2,000 units per day. Because vitamin D is a fat-soluble vitamin, it's best absorbed when you take it with food. You can take it in divided amounts during the day with food.

✔ If your levels are lower than 40 ng/mL, you may need to increase your dose of vitamin D_3 until your levels are up to par. This can mean an average of 3,000 to 5,000 units per day.

✔ Vitamin D can increase the absorption of calcium and phosphorous, so I tend to check calcium levels on anyone for whom I increase vitamin D dosage. If a person has kidney stones or has a problem with high calcium levels, vitamin D_3 may not be appropriate — or it should be used at very low doses.

Eyeing vitamin E

There are eight basic forms of vitamin E, including the tocotrienols and the tocopherols. A good vitamin E supplement should contain all eight to provide the maximum benefit. I tend to start people with a dose of 200 milligrams a day. You usually take a vitamin E capsule with food for maximum absorption.

Kicking it with vitamin K

Vitamin K has several important functions. It promotes the health of both the bones and the blood vessels by inhibiting the leaching of calcium from the bones and preventing the influx of calcium into the blood vessels.

If you're taking warfarin (Coumadin) for treatment of a heart arrhythmia, a clot in the veins of the leg *(deep venous thrombosis),* or a clot in the lungs *(pulmonary embolism),* do not take vitamin K_2. It can affect the liver's processing of warfarin and have a life-threatening interaction.

I (coauthor Rich) tend to start vitamin K_2 at doses of 40 micrograms a day and increase to 60 micrograms over time. This vitamin is taken once a day. Because vitamin K_2 is fat-soluble, it has a better absorption rate when you take it with food.

Providing Energy to Your Cells

All your cells, including the cells of your adrenal glands, need energy to do their job. Vitamins are an important part of the equation, but they aren't the whole answer. You should consider other supplements as well.

For your cells to perform optimally, your mitochondria (the power centers of the cell) need to be powered up. Here are a few supplements that can help in this regard:

- Alpha lipoic acid
- Carnitine
- D-ribose
- Iodine
- Pyrroloquinoline quinone (PQQ)
- Ubiquinone (coenzyme Q_{10})

These supplements are available at your local health food store. You can start most of them, except for iodine, without prior testing.

Adding alpha lipoic acid

There's no better antioxidant for the cell than alpha lipoic acid (ALA). By helping the cell regenerate *glutathione,* which is the most potent cell antioxidant, ALA helps fight oxidative stress and free-radical formation. It also helps the cell regenerate other antioxidants, including vitamins C and E. A stressed adrenal gland needs all the vitamin C it can get!

ALA also helps the body normalize blood glucose levels. If the blood glucose levels are higher than normal (as can happen with excess cortisol secretion associated with adrenal fatigue), ALA can help lower blood glucose.

An ALA supplement is a pill that you take orally, usually in divided doses twice a day. I (coauthor Rich) recommend starting ALA at a lower dose, approximately 200 milligrams a day, and increasing the dose very slowly, because a side effect of ALA can be low sugar levels. I try to aim for at least 400 to 600 milligrams a day if possible.

Do energy drinks really provide energy?

You turn on the television and can't help but see commercials of people falling asleep at their desks. After they take an energy drink or pop an energy pill, they seem to be productive and full of energy, ready to take on the rest of their day.

Do energy drinks provide much-needed energy? On the contrary, they tend to overwork the adrenal glands big time. You get a burst of hormones produced by the adrenal glands, including epinephrine, norepinephrine, and cortisol — only to crash later. The energy drinks can easily overwork the adrenal glands and hasten the development of adrenal fatigue. Eating a candy bar to get the quick sugar rush does a similar thing. For people who already have adrenal fatigue, energy drinks are the worst thing you can take.

Choosing carnitine

Carnitine, a substance produced by the kidneys, is decreased in adrenal fatigue. With chronic illness, carnitine supplementation can help provide energy to the cells. Carnitine is usually taken in pill form, usually 1 to 2 grams in divided doses throughout the day.

Rockin' it with D-ribose

D-ribose is one of the best supplements to help provide your cells with the energy they need to perform optimally. Ribose is a natural sugar and is one of the building blocks of adenosine-5'-triphosphate (ATP), which is the fundamental unit of energy transfer for the cell.

I (coauthor Rich) highly recommend D-ribose supplements. Ribose is necessary for ATP to keep the adrenal cells functioning optimally. Here are three key points about D-ribose supplementation:

✔ You can commonly get D-ribose in capsule or powdered form. I prefer the powdered form because it's easy to take in large doses. A common powdered form can provide 2,500 milligrams per teaspoon. I tend to start a patient with this amount and ask him or her to increase it in a few weeks. A maximum total dose is usually 10,000 to 15,000 milligrams per day. Most people put the powder in their morning drink.

✔ A potential side effect of D-ribose supplements is diarrhea, which is usually dose-dependent. That's why I tend to begin a patient at a lower dose and increase slowly.

✔ Although ribose is a natural sugar, it doesn't tend to increase blood glucose levels. If you have diabetes, this supplement is okay to take.

D-ribose is excellent not only for adrenal fatigue but also for overlapping syndromes, including fibromyalgia and chronic fatigue syndrome.

Investigating iodine

Iodine is a mineral that's necessary for normal cellular function. When people think of iodine deficiency, they commonly think of the thyroid gland. (An iodine deficiency produces a *goiter,* a swelling of the thyroid gland.) Guess what! The adrenal glands need iodine, too. The hypothalamic-pituitary-adrenal axis (HPA axis) likely requires iodine for optimal functioning.

Over time, low levels of iodine may affect the ability of the adrenal glands to produce cortisol. In a lab-based study from the *Journal of Neuroendocrinology* published in 2003, rats were fed an iodine-deficient diet for 6 months. The researchers compared the normal and stress-induced levels of cortisol secretion to those of animals that simply had low thyroid function. The authors noted that the iodine-deficient animals had a loss of the normal daily secretion of cortisol, compared to the other group. They also found that the rats with the low iodine levels, when subjected to a stressor, were unable to mount a similar stress-induced cortisol response, compared to the other group. Even when these animals (who were iodine-deficient for 6 months) were given an iodine-rich diet, their levels of cortisol secretion were reduced.

If you think about these results in the context of adrenal fatigue, low iodine levels may increase the risk of developing adrenal exhaustion earlier, as the adrenal glands aren't able to meet the demands of a stressor.

You may be at more of a risk for iodine deficiency than you think. Environmental toxins, such as the chlorine and fluorine in water and bromine in many household products, can affect your body's ability to absorb iodine. If you have adrenal fatigue, it's a good idea to have your iodine levels checked and take supplements if needed.

Pressing on with pyrroloquinoline quinone

Pyrroloquinoline quinone (PQQ for short) is an important catalyst for a number of chemical reactions in the body. PQQ supplements not only provide a boost to the mitochondria of the cells but also function as free-radical scavengers, eating up all the free radicals. PQQ also protects the brain and boosts cognition. If you have brain fog connected with adrenal fatigue,

PQQ should be part of your arsenal. In a lab-based study from the journal *Neurochemical Research* in 2013, PQQ was found to decrease the formation of *glutamate,* which is a potent neurotoxin.

Your body doesn't make PQQ, so you need to consume it on a daily basis. Foods that are high in PQQ include beans and fruits and vegetables, such as green peppers, papaya, and yams. Green tea is also a great source of PQQ.

Different formulations of PQQ supplements are available. PQQ comes in a pill form that you can take once daily. Start at 10 milligrams a day. Another option is to take PQQ in combination with coenzyme Q_{10} once daily (see the next section).

Utilizing ubiquinone (coenzyme Q_{10})

In chronic illness, especially adrenal fatigue, the levels of ubiquinone (coenzyme Q_{10}) can be low. You need optimal levels of this enzyme not only to help provide energy to the mitochondria but also to help the cell deal with oxidative stress and the free radicals that form in the setting of inflammation and chronic illness. The main dietary source of ubiquinone is fish, namely salmon.

I (coauthor Rich) strongly encourage people with adrenal fatigue or any chronic condition to supplement with ubiquinone. Here are some general considerations when you use this supplement, which comes in a pill form:

- ✔ I tend to start patients with smaller doses to be taken multiple times during the day. I usually start at 50 milligrams twice a day. My goal is to start ubiquinone early to provide enough reserves before a person develops adrenal exhaustion.

- ✔ If a patient is on medications that may cause ubiquinone depletion, I usually start at doses of 100 milligrams twice a day. Examples of these meds include the statin class of medications (atorvastatin [Lipitor], for example) and beta blockers.

- ✔ Ubiquinone can lower your blood pressure and blood glucose levels, so you need to follow those levels closely. In the setting of adrenal fatigue (especially in the latter stages), if your blood pressure or blood glucose levels are very low, your healthcare provider may discuss decreasing the dose or stopping it entirely.

Reducing Inflammation and Providing Antioxidant Support to Your Cells

An important aspect of the treating adrenal fatigue is combating inflammation. To do so, I (coauthor Rich) recommend that everyone take a strong antioxidant daily. If you eat a healthy diet, do you really need to take an antioxidant? In my opinion, the answer is *yes*. The food you're consuming may not be as nutritious as you think. The soil where many vegetables grow is nutrient-depleted. Add to this the use of genetically modified organisms (GMOs) and preservatives and the toxins in some foods, and you're likely not providing your body with all the nutrition (and antioxidants) that you think that you are.

I tell patients this: If you live in a bubble, you're not subject to any stress, you haven't been diagnosed with any chronic medical condition, you're getting 7 hours of quality sleep each night, and you eat nothing artificial or processed, then you don't need to add a daily antioxidant to your regimen. Unfortunately, no one meets those criteria.

You're likely to underestimate the degree of daily stresses and toxins that your body is exposed to and has to deal with — acidity, oxidative stress, and free-radical formation. I believe that your body needs antioxidant support to deal with these daily stresses.

In this section, you read about different antioxidants to add to your regimen in order to combat inflammation. The supplements are available at your local health food store. No testing is required before starting these supplements, but be sure to consult with your healthcare provider concerning whether the supplements in this section are appropriate for your situation.

Connecting with carotenoids

When you walked through the farmers' market or the produce department at the supermarket, you likely noticed the vibrant colors of many of the vegetables — red, yellow, and green bell peppers; orange carrots; yellow squash. The colors come from carotenoids, the pigments found in many vegetables.

Carotenoids, which include alpha-carotene, beta-carotene, lutein, astaxanthin, and zeaxanthin, have many beneficial properties. The carotenoids are potent antioxidants, and they inhibit certain pathways of inflammation, including the cyclooxygenase pathway.

In the body, some of the highest levels from this group of antioxidants are found in the adrenal glands. Because your body is unable to produce carotenoids, you need to either consume them in the diet or obtain them from supplements. I recommend this class of antioxidants for anyone with adrenal fatigue.

Foods high in carotenoids include pigmented fruits and vegetables, including berries, peppers, and green leafy vegetables. If you're able to get three to four servings of fruits and vegetables a day, you're likely getting an adequate amount of carotenoids. In the setting of adrenal fatigue, I'd supplement with at least 5 milligrams of astaxanthin, 2 milligrams of zeaxanthin, and 5 milligrams of lutein.

Drinking green tea

Green tea is an antioxidant with many health benefits. Research demonstrates that green tea may be especially helpful for combating brain fog associated with adrenal fatigue. The main ingredient in green tea is (get ready for some chemistry) *epigallocatechin gallate (EGCG)*.

An article from the journal *Life Sciences* in 2013 reviewed the anti-inflammatory properties of EGCG in rheumatoid arthritis (RA). This condition, which is strongly associated with inflammation, is a cause of increased adrenal stress and adrenal fatigue. The authors felt that not only was EGCG beneficial in decreasing inflammation associated with rheumatoid arthritis, but EGCG also had heart protective effects.

Green tea is such an excellent antioxidant that you should aim to consume it at least two to three times a day if you can. You can have an 8-ounce cup of green tea with each meal. The amount of caffeine in green tea is very small compared to other caffeinated beverages. If you don't like the taste of the drink, another option is a green tea capsule, which you can take once daily in the morning.

Taking up with turmeric

Turmeric — it's not just for South Asian cooking anymore! Actually, turmeric is a powerful antioxidant that has been used for centuries for its ability to reduce inflammation and treat pain. It's well known in traditional Indian medicine, which is called Ayurveda.

The main ingredient in turmeric is *curcumin,* a substance with powerful anticancer properties and excellent heart benefits. Some laboratory research data strongly suggests that curcumin directly benefits the adrenal glands.

In a study appearing in *Brain Research* in 2005, animals were subjected to daily stress for a period of 3 weeks. Researchers found that the chronic stress increased the thickness of the adrenal glands. The animals also demonstrated increased cortisol levels. The authors found that giving the animals curcumin reversed these changes to the adrenal glands. Because of its strong anti-inflammatory properties, turmeric may decrease the stress on the adrenal glands and subsequently decrease the cortisol production.

Here are two easy ways that you can add turmeric to your diet:

- ✔ **Sprinkle turmeric powder (a spice) on each meal.** Turmeric is in all major grocery stores. (Also see Chapter 14 for a great fruit-and-veggie juice you can make with fresh turmeric.)
- ✔ **Take turmeric capsules.** A typical starting dose is 400 to 500 milligrams a day, taken in the morning. You can buy the capsules at co-ops, at health food stores, or online.

Including quercetin

Quercetin is an antioxidant that has strong anti-inflammatory properties. An article from the *Journal of Research in Medical Sciences* in 2012 demonstrated that quercetin was effective in decreasing C-reactive protein (CRP) and inter-leukin 6 (IL-6) in human subjects. High levels of CRP and IL-6 are suggestive of active inflammation. Quercetin is a strong antioxidant, and it counters the oxidative stress and cellular damage associated with chronic inflammation.

Quercetin can be a tremendous aid if you have any medical conditions affecting the lungs, including asthma, chronic obstructive pulmonary disease (COPD), cystic fibrosis, and bronchiectasis.

Quercetin is a plant pigment found in fruits (apples and berries), vegetables (broccoli and green leafy vegetables), and grains. The trouble is that these foods don't contain much quercetin, so you're probably not getting enough of it in your diet. The answer, in this case, is supplementation. I (coauthor Rich) tend to recommend supplements that have both turmeric and quercetin.

Turmeric and quercetin are called *flavonoids*. Other flavonoids include green tea extract, grape seed extract, pine bark extract, and citrus bioflavonoids. All of them have excellent antioxidant effects, and I like using a supplement complex that contains many of them. You can find many different formulations of bioflavonoid complexes, and each formulation has different amounts of each component. Speak with your healthcare provider to find out which formulation may be appropriate for you.

Looking at low-dose naltrexone

An exciting new avenue for treating inflammation is *low-dose naltrexone (LDN)*. What's remarkable about LDN is how it works: It affects the pain receptors (also called the *opiate receptors*) in the body. Traditionally, this medication was used in treating narcotic overdose. At very low doses, naltrexone has proven very helpful in reducing the level of inflammation in tissues and organs. That's why LDN has been used in the management of Crohn's disease, multiple sclerosis, and other inflammatory and autoimmune conditions.

This medication also helps reduce pain levels. LDN has proven to be very effective for the treatment of chronic pain in fibromyalgia syndrome (FMS). In one randomized trial involving 31 women who were treated with 4.5 milligrams of naltrexone, the treated group reported a significant decrease in pain compared to the untreated group. More research is underway, investigating the role of pain receptor and its connection to reducing inflammation.

A true integrative approach to your health involves looking at all your options, including some prescription medications. At very low doses, naltrexone has virtually no side effects. Most practitioners who prescribe this medication begin low, even as low as 1.5 milligrams, and slowly increase up to 4.5 milligrams over several weeks. If you're suffering from chronic inflammation or from debilitating fibromyalgia pain, consider discussing this option with your healthcare provider. Because of its ability to reduce pain and inflammation, LDN may be very helpful for someone with adrenal fatigue, especially if fibromyalgia is present. Only certain pharmacies prescribe this medication. For more information, go to www.lowdosenaltrexone.org.

Balancing Total Body pH

An important aspect of treating adrenal fatigue is correcting acidosis and balancing total body pH (see Chapter 7 for info on acidosis). In this section, you read about an alkaline-based diet and alkaline water as well as a powder that you can use to keep your body alkaline. Again, be sure to speak with your healthcare practitioner before changing your diet or adding any supplements to your program.

How do you know whether your body pH is too acidic or alkaline? Chapter 5 describes the pH test strips that you can use daily to test your urine pH.

Savoring the alkaline diet

An alkaline diet is essentially a plant-based diet that's rich in fruits and vegetables that have an alkaline pH in the body. The idea is that some foods contribute to total body acidity, and other foods are more alkaline. Many vegetables and citrus fruits are more alkaline.

Alkalinity and cancer

If you have cancer, changing your body pH can have detrimental effects on cancer cells. Not only is acidity a strong driving force for inflammation and adrenal stress, but it also provides an environment that allows cancer cells to survive and flourish. And of course, cancer is one of the greatest stresses on the adrenal glands. This is where bicarbonate replacement can help.

An article in *Cancer Research* in 2009 reviewed the physiology of pH and cancer, looking at mouse models of cancer. The investigators found that not only did treatment with oral

sodium bicarbonate increase the pH (going in the alkaline direction) of cancer cells, but it also decreased the tendency of the cancer cells to spread.

Bicarbonate supplementation can also help treat the pain of cancer. In an article from the *Journal of Pain and Palliative Care Chemotherapy* in 2009, patients who were diagnosed with metastatic prostate cancer were given a form of sodium bicarbonate intravenously. In a 3-month follow-up, all 18 individuals reported a significant improvement in quality of life and overall symptoms, including pain relief.

Although citrus fruits contain citric acid, they have an alkaline effect on the body after they're digested.

Drinking alkaline water

Your body is over 70 percent water. The cells of your body are bathed in water, so the type of water you drink makes a difference. Consuming alkaline water has several benefits, including the following:

- ✔ Increasing the mobility of the gastrointestinal tract and increasing nutrient absorption
- ✔ Aiding in flushing toxins out of the body
- ✔ Preserving kidney function over time
- ✔ Decreasing total body inflammation by normalizing body pH
- ✔ Strengthening bones, keeping them healthy, and helping to buffer the effects of acid buildup on the bones over time

When you buy alkaline water, look for water with a pH of 9 to 9.5. It should be mineralized; that is, the water should contain mineral salts that are found in bone, including magnesium and calcium. These alkaline salts serve as buffers to excess acid so your body doesn't draw the minerals from the bone itself. If you want to buy an alkaline water system, talk with your healthcare provider about which system is right for you.

How much water should you drink? In general, unless you're on some sort of fluid restriction, aim to consume approximately 2 to 3 liters (2.1 to 3.2 quarts) of alkaline water per day. Common reasons your healthcare practitioner may prescribe a fluid restriction include congestive heart failure, kidney disease, and liver disease.

Going gaga over greens powder

Test your pH first thing in the morning. Why? If your urine pH is low (that is, less than 6.5), you need to take something alkaline in the morning. Options include an 8-ounce glass of alkaline water (see the preceding section), juice from fresh vegetables and fruits (see Chapter 14 for information on juicing), and greens powder.

Many types of greens powders are available. The powder you choose should have a large amount of plant-based nutrients and antioxidant support. Two greens powders that I (coauthor Rich) really like are Barlean's Greens and Lifetime's Life's Basics Plant Protein with Greens. I take a half of a scoop of the latter first thing in the morning in an 8-ounce glass of alkaline water. I try to take another dose later in the day. The greens powder contains nutrients and antioxidants that are alkaline and can balance your pH. If your greens powder doesn't contain a scoop (or if you can't find it), then just add two heaping tablespoons to an 8-ounce glass of water and drink up.

A greens powder is also a great way to make up for those vegetables that you may not be eating. Taking a scoop of greens powder in the morning can compensate for those servings you're likely not consuming at lunch.

Normalizing Intestinal Health

Don't pass over this section on intestinal health. You'll never decrease the stress on the adrenal glands if you don't bring your intestine back into balance. (In Chapter 8, you see how problems in the gut contribute to adrenal fatigue.) Here are three important techniques for normalizing/improving intestinal health:

- ✔ Consuming probiotics
- ✔ Taking digestive enzymes
- ✔ Fighting fungal overgrowth

Before you start the following supplements, be sure to check with your healthcare provider to see which ones are appropriate in your situation.

Probing probiotics

It's virtually impossible to go into a store or watch television without seeing an advertisement about probiotics. *Probiotics* are live bacteria that you consume to improve your health. In essence, they're used to put the beneficial bacteria back in the intestine to help normalize the intestinal flora. (Please refer to Chapter 8 for a discussion of the importance of intestinal flora to total body health.)

Probiotic supplements can come in many formulations. The few that I (coauthor Rich) frequently use are in capsule form; they're easily digested and tolerated.

You know that probiotics are important. The big question is what you should look for. You need to read the ingredients on each container before you buy. Here are three things to consider:

- ✔ **The number of colony-forming units (CFUs):** The higher the number, the better. Note that there are trillions of organisms in your intestine, so the colony-forming units should be in the billions at least.

- ✔ **The types of organisms that are in your probiotic:** A good probiotic should have a variety of species, including *Lactobacillus acidophilus* and *Bifidobacterium* species. Also look for brands that have *Saccharomyces boulardii.*

- ✔ **Storage considerations:** Some brands of probiotics need to be refrigerated. Others can be kept at room temperature.

Your local health food store will have many different brands of probiotics. Read the directions on the labels concerning when and how often to take them. Some can be taken only on an empty stomach; others, only with meals. Many, if not all, are in a capsule form that can be taken two to three times a day.

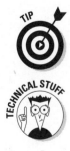

If you've been prescribed an antibiotic, take the probiotic a few hours after the antibiotic. If you take them at the same time, the antibiotic may kill the beneficial bacteria in the probiotic. The idea behind the probiotic is that it decreases the risk of developing antibiotic-associated inflammation of the colon as well as *Clostridium difficile* colitis (see Chapter 8).

Probiotics are also in the following foods:

- ✔ Yogurt, cheese, and kefir (a yogurt-type drink)
- ✔ Unpasteurized sauerkraut
- ✔ Kimchi (a cabbage mix in Korean foods)
- ✔ Miso (as in the Japanese soup)

Prebiotics: Feeding the good bacteria

Prebiotics are food ingredients that feed the probiotics to help them thrive. Prebiotics are in the following foods:

- Chicory root (now added into a lot of foods to provide fiber, called *inulin*)
- Jerusalem artichoke
- Dandelion greens
- Garlic, leeks, and onions
- Bran and oats (raw)
- Plantains or slightly green bananas

Prebiotic compounds are now found in foods that are being touted as *functional foods*. There's no need to get wrapped up in that term, but be familiar with these compounds in case you see them on food labels:

- **FOS:** Fructooligosaccharides
- **GOS:** Galactooligosaccharides
- **XOS:** Xylooligosaccharides
- **Inulin:** Inulin (a group of polysaccharides); this is a popular addition to many food products to provide fiber

Breaking down nutrients with digestive enzymes

If you have *intestinal dysbiosis* (a general term that refers to an unhealthy intestine; see Chapter 8), you're likely not digesting and absorbing the nutrients from your food well due to an imbalance of intestinal bacteria. Digestive enzymes can help your body properly digest the food until you can restore the balance in your intestinal ecosystem.

An enzyme supplement usually consists of various enzymes, including bromelain and papain. You should take the enzyme supplement, which comes in pill form, with each meal. The dosage can vary, so talk with your healthcare practitioner about which digestive enzymes may be suitable for your health situation.

Taking a digestive enzyme before you begin to eat is a no-no — it can cause stomach discomfort. Most people should take digestive enzymes during meals or right after eating.

Fighting fungal overgrowth

Treating intestinal dysbiosis involves eradicating *Candida* (a yeast) from the intestine. You can use several supplements to help eliminate *Candida;* they also have other health benefits.

✔ **Oil of oregano:** This oil is a natural preparation for eliminating yeast from your intestine. It's also a natural antibiotic, effective against many common bacterial pathogens. Oil of oregano comes in various forms, including softgels and straight oil. Depending on the brand of the oil of oregano, the dosage can vary.

✔ **Garlic:** Garlic isn't just an excellent supplement for eliminating *Candida*. It also protects your blood vessels, helping to keep them soft and pliable. It's a potent antioxidant, and it's excellent for treating high cholesterol.

The form of garlic that you want to take is *aged garlic extract,* which comes in capsule form. You can begin with a dose of 400 to 600 milligrams a day, usually once a day.

Garlic is a natural blood thinner, so if you're on blood-thinning medication such as aspirin, clopidogrel (Plavix), or warfarin (Coumadin), talk to your healthcare provider before starting aged garlic extract.

✔ **Olive leaf extract:** Olive leaf extract is a potent antifungal agent. A recommended starting dose is 500 milligrams a day, taken once a day.

Because olive leaf extract can lower blood pressure, you need to talk with your healthcare provider before starting this extract. You also need to monitor your blood pressure on a daily basis when taking this supplement.

✔ **Grape seed extract:** Not only does this extract have potent antioxidant properties, but it also has excellent *Candida*-killing properties. Grape seed extract capsules should be taken at least once a day at a dose of 250 milligrams.

✔ **Coconut oil:** Coconut oil has antifungal properties. I (coauthor Rich) like softgels, and I ask people to try to consume at least 1,000 milligrams of this supplement per day. Some people enjoy just eating the coconut oil, 1 to 2 tablespoons daily.

Oil of oregano, olive leaf extract, and grape seed extract can kill both good and bad bacteria, so take them in moderation, as directed by your healthcare provider. Also make sure you take *Candida*-killing supplements separately from probiotics (discussed earlier in "Probing probiotics"). Taking them at the same time as probiotics diminishes the probiotics' effectiveness in re-establishing normal bowel flora.

A common practice is rotating the supplements you use for eradicating *Candida*. Every practitioner is different, but some rotate their antifungal regimens on a 1- to 2-week interval. The idea is to decrease the risk that the *Candida* will develop resistance to one anti-yeast regimen. By using various antifungal agents on a varied schedule, you're more apt to eradicate the yeast.

If you don't eliminate sugar from your diet, the *Candida*-killing supplements won't be as effective. Sugar is a potent stimulus for yeast overgrowth (that's what yeast eats); consuming sugar is like adding fuel to a fire.

Getting Some Sleep with the Help of Supplements

One of the biggest problems that someone with adrenal fatigue has is getting a good night's sleep (see Chapter 6). Here are some supplements you can take to help you rest:

- ✔ **Melatonin:** Your body normally secretes the hormone melatonin at night as part of your sleep-wake cycle. If you have adrenal fatigue, your body likely produces less melatonin than it should at night. Supplementation with melatonin may improve your quality of sleep.

  Start at low doses of 1 to 2 milligrams of melatonin each night before going to sleep (or trying to go to sleep) and increase slowly. The highest dose that I (coauthor Rich) usually prescribe is 10 milligrams. Other practitioners may use higher doses.

- ✔ **Valerian root:** Valerian is an herb. In one insomnia study, researchers noted that although further study was needed, valerian root seemed to improve the quality of sleep without causing any significant side effects.

  Although different brands vary, an average dosage of valerian root is 1,000 to 1,500 milligrams. I tend to recommend the capsule form because it's very easy to swallow and well-tolerated. You can take it approximately 1 hour prior to going to bed.

- ✔ **L-theanine:** L-theanine is an amino acid that inhibits the action of glutamate (a very toxic substance) in the brain. A few studies have demonstrated its efficacy in helping people get a good night's sleep. It's also a great stress reliever. You can start doses of L-theanine at 50 to 100 milligrams a night.

Of course, before taking any of these supplements, speak with your healthcare provider to see whether they're appropriate for you.

Considering prescription sleep aids

With adrenal fatigue, getting a good night's sleep is often a struggle, so people often ask whether they should consider prescription sleep aids. My answer is *yes*, if needed. The key is to discuss some of the side effects of sleep medication with your healthcare provider. The most common prescription sleep aids include a class of medications called benzodiazepines; this class includes diazepam (Valium) and alprazolam (Xanax). Another commonly prescribed medication is zolpidem (Ambien).

Benzodiazepines are effective in helping someone get a good night's sleep, but be aware of potential side effects:

✔ **Paradoxical excitation:** Instead of causing someone to go asleep, they can cause the opposite: The person may become excitable and unable to sleep.

✔ **Confusion and lethargy:** These side effects are more common in the elderly, so I tend to minimize the use of the benzodiazepines in the elderly population.

Be aware that many of the benzodiazepines depend on having the liver process them. If you have liver disease or cirrhosis, the benzodiazepine doses need to be substantially reduced, or another medication needs to be chosen, because reduced liver function means these medications can stay in the body for a long period of time.

Using Stronger Herbs for a Major Boost

This section brings out some of the big guns — herbs that can provide the adrenal glands with the boost they need when you're dealing with adrenal fatigue and especially with adrenal exhaustion. I (coauthor Rich) often recommend adding these to your regimen when the symptoms of adrenal fatigue either don't abate or worsen (see Chapter 4 for the symptoms). Many of the items in this section also help to reduce the effects of stress.

The following herbs are called *adaptogens,* which are plants that practitioners of herbal medicine believe decrease cellular sensitivity to stress. These herbs help restore balance not only to the adrenal glands but also to the entire body. They help the adrenal glands cope with the stress response, partly by de-stressing the adrenal glands and partly by providing a boost to adrenal gland function. Again, before you start the following herbs, you should check in with your healthcare provider to see whether they may be helpful for you.

Think of the herbs in this section as providing a major tune-up to fatigued adrenal glands, allowing your body to run better and more efficiently.

Assessing ashwagandha

Ashwaghanda *(Withania somnifera)* is an herb that can improve your response to stress. Over the centuries (yes, it's been used in Ayurvedic medicine for centuries), people have viewed ashwagandha as a substance that helps the body rejuvenate itself.

An interesting study published in the *Indian Journal of Psychological Medicine* in 2012 enrolled approximately 60 individuals who had a clinical history of being chronically stressed. Half the participants received a placebo, and the other half was treated with a dose of 300 milligrams of ashwagandha daily. Those who were treated with this herb noticed an improvement in overall quality of life and in how they responded to stress, as evaluated through stress-assessment questionnaires. Those treated with ashwagandha showed a substantial decrease in stress scores when compared to the placebo group. The investigators also noted another important finding: The blood levels of cortisol were lower in the group treated with ashwagandha than in the control group. Ashwagandha appeared to provide a boost that the adrenal glands needed.

Ashwagandha is available in several forms, including root and extract forms. I (coauthor Rich) tend to recommend the capsule form of this herb. An average dose is approximately 500 to 600 milligrams, depending on the brand. To start, take this herb once a day, and after 3 to 4 weeks, you can increase the dose to twice a day.

Evaluating eleuthero

Eleuthero *(Eleutherococcus senticosus),* formerly referred to as *Siberian ginseng,* is a great herb that can help improve the adrenal glands' response to stress. It helps boost the function of the adrenal glands. Eleuthero has also been shown to help boost the immune system. And here's a bonus: It's helpful in improving cognition.

Eleuthero can be taken in capsule form or in liquid form. I (coauthor Rich) tend to use the capsule form, for which a usual dose is 400 to 500 milligrams once a day, depending on the brand.

On a personal note, I noticed an improvement since I began taking eleuthero. I began taking a 450-milligram capsule once a day. I was less stressed, had more energy, and felt calmer throughout the day.

Loving licorice

Licorice (also known as *glycyrrhizic acid*) is commonly recommended for treating *hypotension* (low blood pressure) in adrenal fatigue. Hypotension often occurs in the latter stages of adrenal fatigue, and licorice can be a tremendous help.

Licorice is available in capsule form. The recommended dosage is approximately 1 to 2 grams in divided doses, taken twice a day.

Because licorice can cause too little potassium *(hypokalemia),* your healthcare practitioner needs to follow your potassium levels, which can be done with a simple blood test.

Don't use licorice if you have high blood pressure *(hypertension);* use it only if your blood pressure is low or if you experience dizziness when standing up (a sign of orthostatic hypotension). Talk with your healthcare practitioner if you have any heart problems. Given the risk of low potassium and licorice's potential interaction with heart medications, including digoxin, you may need to avoid licorice if you have any heart problems.

Reeling it in with Rhodiola

Rhodiola is a genus of herbs that's beneficial not only for reducing stress and boosting adrenal function but also for improving sleep quality.

A study from the journal *Planta Medica* in 2009 evaluated the effects of *Rhodiola* on reducing stress and fatigue. Sixty individuals were divided into two groups; one group received a placebo, and another received *Rhodiola*. The study participants were followed for 4 weeks. At the end of the study, the participants who had taken *Rhodiola* reported increased endurance, increased mental clarity, and a better ability to concentrate on tasks. The researchers also noted that the *Rhodiola* group had decreased cortisol levels when compared to those in the placebo group.

Rhodiola comes in several forms, but I (coauthor Rich) recommend the capsule form. An average starting dose is 400 milligrams a day, usually taken before a meal.

Exercising care with adrenal glandular extract

Adrenal extracts are used to help restore the adrenal function to normal. They're usually made from the adrenal cortex of other animals. For example, *bovine adrenal extract* comes from cows. These extracts are usually used for only a short period of time, until adrenal function is restored.

You can purchase many adrenal glandular extracts in tablet or capsule form. An average dosing for the adrenal glandular extract is 100 to 200 milligrams, depending on the brand. The extract is usually taken two to three times a day.

Warning: Because adrenal glandular extract comes from the adrenal glands of animals (especially cows), using this extract offers a slight risk of obtaining *bovine spongiform encephalopathy (BSE),* which can be fatal in humans. You need to be sure that you obtain your glandular extracts only from a reputable company. Please talk with your healthcare practitioner before purchasing a glandular extract.

Detoxifying

One important aspect of adrenal fatigue treatment is detoxification. The contaminants and heavy metals in the water supply and the chemicals and pesticides in foods are examples of toxins everyone is likely to consume on a daily basis. Most people aren't even aware of these toxins. Toxin buildup can increase stress and make you lethargic and exhausted.

Your healthcare practitioner may recommend a form of detoxification as part of your treatment for adrenal fatigue, especially if some of the testing that you've had done demonstrates that your body has a high toxic load (see Chapter 5 for info on hair testing). Above and beyond the specific results of any test, the toxins that you're exposed to daily can worsen adrenal stress. You and your healthcare provider should consider detoxification as part of your treatment plan for adrenal fatigue.

I (coauthor Rich) worry that rapid detoxification methods will overstress already-exhausted adrenal glands. I also worry about the risks of dehydration and electrolyte imbalances. A slower type of detoxification is a better option. You're at lower risk of dehydration, and the program is generally well-tolerated.

Understand that in detoxification, you may feel worse before you feel better, because the toxins in the body tissues need to enter the bloodstream so they can be eliminated by the kidneys. You may need to have blood work done before, during, and after the detoxification process to assess your electrolyte status and kidney function.

If you're considering undergoing detoxification, do so under the supervision of a healthcare practitioner. Here are some of my general principles for detoxification:

- ✔ I use alkaline water as my base. Consume at least 2 to 3 liters on a daily basis. (See the earlier section "Drinking alkaline water.")

- ✔ I tend to supplement with antioxidants, minerals, and vitamins through-out the day, including green tea extract, a greens powder, vitamins C and B_5, and an antioxidant complex such as a carotenoid. Your health-care practitioner may recommend other antioxidants and supplements during the detoxification process.

- ✔ I believe that making and drinking juice in the morning (as detailed in Chapter 14) is a great way to start off a detox.

- ✔ I take probiotics twice daily. (See the earlier section "Probing probiotics.")

Detox plans are different; a slow detox plan for someone with adrenal fatigue can last for 1 to 2 months. After that, your healthcare provider will likely develop a personalized maintenance plan for you that will include probiotics and a combination of nutrients and antioxidants.

If you have kidney disease, heart disease, or diabetes, your detox plan needs to be altered accordingly. For example, if you have a history of coronary heart failure (CHF), your fluid intake may need to be restricted. With diabetes, your blood glucose levels need to be monitored closely.

Chapter 12

Exercising and Eating the Right Way

....

....

*E*xercise has many benefits, including increased endurance, increased muscle strength, and improved flexibility. It also protects your heart. But if you have adrenal fatigue, exercising the *wrong way* can make you feel more tired and may even create an energy crisis that's difficult to recover from. Exercising the *right way* improves the adrenal glands' ability to deal with stress and helps them work more efficiently.

Bad nutritional practices are a significant cause of adrenal fatigue. As you read in Chapters 8 and 11, your adrenal glands need the right fuel to function optimally. Changing your eating habits to include whole foods that have high nutritional value is vital to restoring adrenal health, especially if you're going to begin an exercise program.

In this chapter, you discover the basics of exercising safely. You also look at types of exercise, find out how to eat well before a workout, and get the scoop on helping your body repair itself if you do too much too fast. We wrap up with a basic approach to finding, preparing, eating, and enjoying the right foods.

Before you embark on any exercise program, talk with your healthcare provider to determine which types of exercise are safe for you to do. After you obtain medical clearance, be sure to speak to a certified and licensed trainer (if your state licenses trainers). People often go to the gym and work out on various machines without having a definite program in mind, and they're the people who hurt themselves and stop exercising.

Staying Safe as You Exercise

For all athletic activity, you always want to do a few things for safety's sake. The list includes warming up, monitoring your vital signs during your workout, and cooling down. These three practices are even more important in the setting of adrenal fatigue. In the beginning, don't even think about working out without having a way to monitor your blood pressure.

Warming up and stretching

Before beginning any workout, you need to prepare your muscles for exercise. Warming up properly is important for a couple of reasons:

- ✔ It prepares your muscles for a higher level of intensity, which is especially important in adrenal fatigue. Warming up adequately decreases your risk of developing muscle fatigue.

- ✔ It reduces the risk of injury to your muscles.

In most cases, if you spend a little time doing some light aerobic work, such as walking, biking against light resistance, or light jogging, that's enough to get the blood flowing to your muscles. You should warm up for at least 20 minutes.

If you have fibromyalgia, arthritis, or other joint problems, the warm-up is especially important. With fibromyalgia in particular, the risk of muscle fatigue and muscle pain is much higher if you don't do a proper warm-up.

After warming up, you should stretch for at least 5 minutes. Never stretch a cold muscle, or you increase the risk of injury. At the very least, stretch your quadriceps, hamstrings, and calf muscles. You can find some great pictures and exercise videos that demonstrate proper stretching techniques and exercises at www.bodybuilding.com/fun/bbmaintrain.htm. Another resource for stretching is *Stretching For Dummies* by LaReine Chabut (Wiley).

Monitoring your vital signs

When you exercise, pay attention to your vital signs, mainly your blood pressure and heart rate.

Signs of adrenal fatigue include a lowered blood pressure, so you want to monitor your blood pressure to make sure it doesn't drop when you're exercising. Perspiring causes fluid losses, which can cause a decrease in blood pressure in someone with adrenal fatigue. If you feel dizzy, stop exercising.

You can wear a portable blood pressure cuff on your arm to record your blood pressure and heart rate while you exercise. Many exercise machines (including treadmills and exercise bikes) have built-in monitoring systems that let you track your pulse. In most cases, though, they don't monitor blood pressure, so you'll need to bring your own blood pressure cuff to the gym.

Staying hydrated

No matter what type of exercise you engage in, you're likely to perspire. When you sweat, you lose salt and other electrolytes through the skin. These losses can be critical in someone with adrenal fatigue, because you need salt and electrolytes to help maintain your blood pressure.

To avoid dehydration and electrolyte loss, be sure that you have an electrolyte replacement solution with you when you're exercising. Many of the commercial electrolyte solutions are very high in sugar and have little or no electrolyte replacement value, so we think the best electrolyte solution is one you make yourself. Follow these three steps:

1. **Fill a 15- to 20-ounce water bottle with alkaline water.**

   See Chapter 11 for details on alkaline water.

2. **Add a squeeze of lemon or lime.**

3. **Add ¼ teaspoon Himalayan pink salt or Celtic Sea Salt to this water bottle and mix.**

Cooling down (and stretching again)

The cool-down is just as important as the warm-up. After the workout is over, take 5 to 10 minutes to gradually decrease activity. Why? Because without it, your muscles will cramp up, and they'll be especially tight, painful, and difficult to warm up for your next workout.

A cool-down is nothing special. If you're jogging, walk for 10 minutes and stretch lightly. If you're using weight machines or free weights in a gym, spend a few extra minutes walking at a slower pace on the treadmill or walking a few laps. If you're lifting weights at home, just walk a little.

You also want to gently stretch your muscles after the workout to prevent them from cramping and becoming too sore the next day. Here are two light stretching exercises that you can do quickly and easily:

✔ **Calf stretch:** Stand approximately 1 to 2 feet away from the wall with your feet together. Keep your legs straight and lean toward the wall. Hold your breath for a slow count of four and then return to your starting position. Repeat twice.

✔ **Hamstring stretch:** Find a chair that's approximately knee-high and place your leg on the seat of the chair. Turn your upper body 90 degrees to the opposite side. Try to press your leg into the chair. Hold this stretch for a slow count of four and repeat. Switch and repeat this exercise twice with your other leg.

At Ease: Performing Meditative Exercises

Meditation-based exercises include yoga and t'ai chi (t'ai chi ch'uan). Yoga is possibly 5,000 years old, and t'ai chi is at least 900 years old. They've lasted because they do people good. These exercises are relatively slow in pace but can still provide quite a workout. They focus on paced and purposeful movements (if you've ever attended a yoga class or t'ai chi lesson, you know what we're talking about). Here are some of the benefits:

✔ These exercises are energy-promoting, not energy-depleting.

✔ They aren't known to cause drops in blood pressure or changes in pulse rate.

✔ They increase muscle strength and endurance.

✔ They can reduce pain and inflammation.

People with adrenal fatigue tolerate meditative exercise very well. We advocate beginning with this type of exercise and then slowly incorporating aerobic and/or muscle resistance training. (We talk about these forms of exercise later in the chapter.) If you have adrenal fatigue, one of the two exercise modalities in this section should be part of your daily regimen.

Incorporating yoga

Yoga is a holistic meditative exercise with roots in India. Like other forms of meditative exercise, it emphasizes concentration and contemplation, deep breathing, and different physical movements. The goal of yoga is not only to treat the physical but also to bring the emotional and spiritual aspects of yourself back into harmony. If there was ever a "healing practice" better suited for the ongoing treatment of adrenal fatigue, we're not sure what that would be.

Many studies report the general health benefits of yoga, and a few demonstrate the benefits for adrenal health. In one 2011 study from the *Journal of the American Academy of Nurse Practitioners,* 18 women who were breast cancer survivors were randomly split into two groups. Nine women were assigned to attend 1½-hour yoga sessions twice a week for approximately 2 months, compared to a control group that received no intervention. An important objective of the study was evaluation of salivary cortisol levels throughout the day. The treatment group demonstrated lower salivary cortisol levels in the morning and in the late afternoon when compared to the control group. And at the end of the study, the women who attended the yoga sessions reported improved energy levels, less depression, and better feelings about themselves and things.

I (coauthor Rich) consider this to be a very important study. Cancer is a known cause of adrenal fatigue and inflammation. I conclude that yoga was able to lower cortisol levels and boost the adrenals. It decreased the workload of the adrenal glands and improved stamina.

Various forms of yoga exist; in the United States, hatha yoga is the best known. You can learn yoga in various ways — by having personalized one-on-one sessions with a yoga instructor (which can be expensive), watching television or instructional yoga videos/DVDs, going to a yoga class, and so on. I recommend going to a class; many of my patients attend yoga classes on a regular basis, and the experiences they've reported to me are fantastic:

- ✔ **The connection with others and the instructor in a group setting is a big plus.** Exercising alone can be isolating, whereas exercising with others can be a great motivator to keep going.

- ✔ **Although you connect with others, you get a sense of personal space and centering that's very important.** The breathing exercises employed at the beginning of most yoga classes are vital in centering yourself and preparing yourself emotionally and physically for the class.

- ✔ **Little or no equipment is needed.** In most cases, all you need is to wear fitted pants and tops that aren't restrictive and to get an inexpensive yoga mat. Oh, and you need to bring your whole self to the class as well.

Yoga can be learned, but figuring it out takes time. You need to be patient. Most yoga centers have beginning classes you attend before going on to the advanced classes. The physical movements associated with yoga become more difficult as you advance through each class, but your ability slowly increases. Give yourself time to start at the beginning and learn (and master) things slowly. There are no shortcuts here. Many of my patients attend yoga at least two to three times a week.

Taking up t'ai chi

T'ai chi (t'ai chi ch'uan) has been practiced in China for centuries. It has a lot in common with yoga, with an emphasis on physical movement, proper breathing to find your core center, and balance between the spirit and the body.

Unlike yoga (where you sit or lie down for part of the practice), you usually stand for t'ai chi. T'ai chi consists of defined body movements that are often described as "flowing." The movements must be learned, but almost anyone can do them, including the elderly and people with some physical limitations. Even a person in a wheelchair can do the arm movements. ***Bonus:*** The moves have great names, such as "White Stork Spreads Wings" and "Carry Tiger to Mountain."

T'ai chi can increase your muscle strength and flexibility and can improve your endurance. It can also boost your immune system, so if you have adrenal fatigue and suffer from repeated infections that you never seem to fully recover from, you should strongly consider t'ai chi.

An interesting study reported in the journal *Diabetes Care* in 2007 examined the effects of t'ai chi on diabetes parameters and immune system health. Diabetes is an example of a chronic illness that causes increased adrenal stress and adrenal fatigue. In this study, a group of 39 people took part in regular t'ai chi sessions over a 12-week period. At the end of the study, 32 had finished, and the researchers noted the following:

- **There was a significant decrease in each participant's glycosylated hemoglobin (A1C) level, which is one way that healthcare practitioners measure diabetes control.** Basically, this number measures how controlled your blood glucose levels are over a 3-month period. The lower the levels, the better the control. Diabetes is defined as an A1C value of 6.6 or higher, so most healthcare practitioners aim for a value below that number.

- **Participants didn't show a significant decrease in random fasting blood glucose levels.** This is a good thing because it means that t'ai chi didn't place people at risk of developing *hypoglycemia* (low blood sugar). Someone with diabetes and/or adrenal fatigue can develop hypoglycemia.

- **T cell levels increased, indicating an improved immune system.** The investigators wanted to assess how the immune system improved by measuring all sorts of T lymphocyte (T cell) functions. T cells are very important in regulating the immune system and fighting off infection. T'ai chi raised the levels of T cells in the body. The better your immune system is functioning, the less stress on the adrenal glands.

A few patients of mine practice t'ai chi regularly. Although some practice in their homes, many choose to attend classes. They find they can more easily do the exercises in a class environment. The result: They feel better and note improved endurance and a better quality of life. Even my elderly patients feel that their ability to get up and move around has improved, thanks to t'ai chi. You should aim to do t'ai chi at least two to three times a week.

Feel the Burn: Enjoying an Aerobic Workout

Aerobic exercise — such as walking and cycling — is the most common type of exercise that people engage in. Aerobic exercises have the following characteristics:

✔ They're long in duration and usually low in intensity. This allows the body to adapt to them over the course of the workout and over time.

✔ The risks of dehydration can increase over the course of the workout.

✔ Over time, they tend to decrease blood pressure and heart rate.

Aerobic exercise tends to be better tolerated than other forms of exercise, including higher intensity anaerobic exercises and muscle resistance training. (You read about these forms of exercise later in this chapter.)

Exercise can deplete the energy in a muscle quickly, so pay attention to your body. With adrenal fatigue, muscle cells' mitochondria may not function optimally, and with some forms of exercise, that may precipitate an energy crisis. Aerobic exercises don't cause an acute energy crisis; however, they tend to cause a cellular energy deficit over time. In other words, exercise can cause muscle pain and extreme muscle fatigue. You literally may not have enough energy to complete the workout.

Enjoying an aerobic workout begins by not inviting pain or fatigue. You can have a lot of fun doing aerobic exercises without much planning or effort. You usually don't need a lot of equipment, but having the proper equipment reduces the risk of injury. In this section, you read about several types of aerobic exercise appropriate for folks with adrenal fatigue.

WARNING!

Anaerobic literally means "without oxygen." This type of exercise is characterized by short, fast, high-intensity bursts; an example is running a 100-meter dash. The muscle fatigue that comes with short-burst, high-intensity exercise can be profound! Someone with adrenal fatigue may take longer to recover from this form of exercise — sometimes as long as a few days. We recommend that you *don't* attempt it as an initial form of exercise. Higher intensity exercise needs to be incorporated into your exercise program slowly; examples appear in the later section "Combining Different Forms of Exercise."

Walking around the block

A couple of miles from where I (coauthor Rich) live, there's a park with a beautiful walking trail about 1 mile long. Nothing's more enjoyable than a brisk walk on a late summer evening or a fall afternoon. Walking is a good initial form of exercise if you have adrenal fatigue because it's very well tolerated compared to other forms of aerobic exercise. It doesn't cause quite as much muscle fatigue as biking or swimming, for example.

Here are some tips concerning walking:

- **Start with a short walk at a normal pace.** Take your first walk at a normal pace and aim for a duration of about 5 to 10 minutes. Then sit down and rest. You may be reading this and thinking, "I feel fine. I know I can do more." Okay, do more a couple of days from now. You have time, so don't push it. With adrenal fatigue, details like that matter.

- **Keep a diary of how you feel after your walk so you can see what works and what doesn't work for you.** See how you feel the day after your first walk. If your first day is too intense, you can crash and burn in the setting of adrenal fatigue.

- **Build gradually.** Instead of walking every day, start out by walking every two to three days. Begin increasing the duration of your walks before you start increasing your pace. In the first few weeks, maintain a normal walking pace and add 30 to 60 seconds to each subsequent walking session. After you're comfortable walking about 30 minutes without stopping or needing to sit down, *then* begin to gradually increase your walking pace.

- **Initially, stay away from hills.** Try to keep your first walking sessions on level ground. More hills means increased muscle soreness the next day.

- **Wear loose-fitting clothes and comfortable footwear.** Sometimes I see people walking around in the park in their work clothes (including dress pants and a shirt), and they don't look comfortable at all.

If you're walking on a treadmill, the same principles apply. Initially, set the machine to a normal walking pace, avoid the hill and interval programs, and wear comfortable clothes and shoes. Consider buying sneakers specifically designed for walking.

If you want to find out how far you walk every day, consider buying a pedometer. It records each step you take. About 2,000 steps is the equivalent of 1 mile.

Enjoying aquatherapy and swimming

Aquatherapy amounts to doing exercises in a pool. Water is great because there's no wear and tear on the joints in the water. In fact, many rehabilitation professionals commonly prescribe aquatherapy to help people recover from a bodily injury or trauma.

Examples of exercises that you can do in the water include walking and running. The water provides resistance, and water-based exercises can help increase muscle strength and flexibility. I (coauthor Rich) am a big proponent of doing aquatherapy first and adding swimming (basically swimming laps) later.

Unless you're going to stay in the shallow end of the pool, wear a life preserver (the fancy term is "personal flotation device") for the first few exercise sessions. If you feel that you're too old for a life preserver, use a life vest or a flotation belt, or exercise with someone else nearby who is available in an emergency. I've seen people with extreme adrenal fatigue become so tired midway through a session that they're unable to continue. You don't want to drown.

Many health clubs, including the YMCA, offer water aerobics classes, which are a combination of endurance and strengthening exercises in a pool. The classes usually range in size from 10 to 20 people. They offer a great opportunity to meet people and socialize as well as exercise!

Although swimming laps is an excellent form of exercise, it can be a bit strenuous initially for someone with adrenal fatigue because it works every muscle group in your upper and lower body. Therefore, make sure you know what your baseline endurance is before you decide to swim laps. One option is to use a kickboard and kick your legs at a low intensity; with a kickboard, you can rest when you need to.

Rowing with light resistance

An oft-forgotten form of aerobic exercise is rowing. One option for this exercise is rowing a boat, which can be peaceful and serene, especially if you do it in the early morning. Another popular option is using a rowing machine or the rowing machine feature of a home gymnasium, such as the Bowflex.

Rowing is great for strengthening your core muscles, including your abdomen and mid to lower back muscles. It also strengthens your leg muscles to some degree, including the quadriceps and hamstrings.

If you're just starting out, I (coauthor Rich) recommend doing sets of 15 to 20 repetitions at a time. Begin with low weight (about 20 pounds of resistance) and gauge how you feel. Start with one set, and after a couple of weeks, increase to doing two sets. Don't row too fast; this isn't the galley battle scene in *Ben Hur!*

Riding a bike

Bicycling is a form of exercise with many variations. Some people feel that it's not a good form of aerobic exercise because you're sitting — you're mainly using your legs, not your upper body. But we think biking is a great workout for folks with adrenal fatigue because you can control your pace, your time, and your level of intensity. For example, if you're riding a bike outside and you want to coast and rest, you can (unless you're going up a hill).

To start, bike a few miles and see how sore and tired your muscles are the next day. If bicycling is new to you, you'll feel it! You can use a road bike, a mountain bike, or a stationary bike. Here are some notes on using a stationary bike:

✔ Bikes that have bigger seats are comfortable to sit on for longer periods of time.

✔ You can read while using the stationary bike, because you don't have to worry about crashing into something or someone. I (coauthor Rich) read medical journals and comic books, but you can read anything and send text messages, too!

Some stationary bikes have moving handlebars that allow you to work your arms as well your legs. The handlebars let you simulate the arm actions of running. Also, some models have a built-in fan that provides cooling relief as you pedal.

Pump It Up: Adding Muscle Resistance Training

The idea of resistance training is to build muscle strength rather than muscle endurance, which you get from aerobic exercise (see the preceding section). Muscle resistance training can use free weights, exercise machines like those at a typical gym, or home machines.

Resistance training should be a component of your overall program for the following reasons:

- ✔ **Studies show that improving muscle strength with resistance training improves bone health.** Over time, high cortisol secretion worsens bone health, and you want to counter those effects. Muscle resistance training increases bone strength and can delay the onset of conditions like osteoporosis.

- ✔ **The excess secretion of cortisol from the adrenal glands can cause muscle atrophy.** Combine this with the fact that many people with adrenal fatigue don't exercise, and the result is muscle groups that haven't really been used in years and need to be strengthened.

- ✔ **Resistance training (especially as people get older) is vital for decreasing the possibility of muscle injury and maintaining functional independence.** You don't want to be driving around the supermarket in a mobility scooter before you absolutely need to.

- ✔ **When you build muscle mass, you increase your metabolism.** An exercised muscle burns calories even after your exercise session is complete.

Muscle resistance training can be either aerobic or anaerobic:

- ✔ **Aerobic:** More repetitions with lower resistance (lighter weights) is a more aerobic form of muscle resistance training. For people with adrenal fatigue, we recommend starting out with lighter weights and fewer reps.

- ✔ **Anaerobic:** In general, fewer repetitions with higher resistance (more pounds of weight) is an anaerobic form of muscle resistance training.

Before starting any muscle resistance program, define your goals. Objectives are typically to improve your overall fitness and increase your muscle strength. Your goal at this point shouldn't be to "get huge." (Don't worry. In time, you'll no doubt be showing firm, well-defined muscles, and you'll probably lose some body fat, too!)

The term *free weights* refers to weights not connected to a machine. When you exercise with free weights such as barbells and dumbbells, you increase the strength, flexibility, and range of motion of your muscles. You're typically exercising more than one of your muscles in more than one way.

Understanding the ways that you move your muscles is important when trying new resistance exercises. A muscle has these basic movements:

✔ **Flexion:** Bending forward, as in bringing your hand to your shoulder

✔ **Extension:** Bending backward, as in extending your hand away from your shoulder

✔ **Abduction:** For example, raising your arm at the side to be level with your shoulder

✔ **Adduction:** For example, lowering your arm to be at your side

✔ **Lateral flexion:** For example, bending to the side

Understanding which muscle groups will be affected in a particular exercise can help you stretch and warm up appropriately (see the earlier section "Warming up and stretching"). For example, some exercises used to strengthen the muscles in the chest work your arms and shoulders as well. Stretching these areas properly is essential to decreasing the risk of muscle fatigue and pain.

Using free weights generally increases your muscle flexibility and range of motion more than doing similar exercises on a machine does. Talk to a trainer about what kinds of exercises are right for you. In general, you should start out doing five to seven repetitions using a weight that you can lift comfortably; then repeat once after a 1- to 2-minute rest. You can increase the number of repetitions with each session.

Weight machines can help you exercise in an efficient way. They're very convenient, and unlike free weights, they don't need to be put back after you've finished your set. One example of an efficient workout is *circuit training*. You do one or two sets of an exercise to work a muscle group and then move to the next machine on the circuit. A typical circuit works the chest, arms, legs, and back. (You can also do this type of workout with free weights.)

If you have adrenal fatigue, we recommend cutting everything in the circuit by 50 percent. Do a half circuit and only half of the repetitions. Start out with five repetitions for each exercise in the circuit and see how you feel. You need to find out what your baseline exercise threshold is. Don't worry. You can gradually make your program more intense.

Before you start any weight training program, pay attention to the following:

✔ **Physical support:** If you're planning to lift anything heavier than 15 pounds for men or 10 pounds for women (and you will be), you need to provide support to your torso and lower back. One way to do this is to use a weight belt. As a bonus, belts look pretty cool at the gym.

✔ **Proper form:** Pay attention to the proper form for each type of exercise. At worst, you risk injury from bad form. At best, you don't work the muscles correctly to get the results you want. Ask one of the trainers at the gym about the form for any weight machine or free weight exercise.

Work with a coach or mentor. You need guidance as to what type of program to follow — which exercises to do, how to use the correct form, how much weight to use, how many repetitions to do in a set, and so forth. Ask the coach about his or her background and education. Note that the term "personal trainer" can mean many things, so be a little skeptical. You don't want someone who just points to a weight machine and says, "Lift that."

Combining Different Forms of Exercise

Doing the same type of exercise over and over can get pretty boring. By mixing it up a bit, you can add variety to your workouts as well as maintain your enthusiasm for exercise. Here are some ways to add variety:

✔ **Combine different forms of aerobic exercise in a workout.** I (coauthor Rich) like to combine rowing and biking in a single workout session. I may start with 30 to 35 repetitions at the rowing machine at moderate resistance, then switch to the stationary bike for a 5-mile bike ride, and then finish with another 30 to 35 reps on the rowing machine.

✔ **Vary the speed or intensity of one type of exercise.** A pure anaerobic workout can cause significant muscle fatigue, and it could cause a muscle energy crisis for someone with adrenal fatigue. However, incorporating anaerobic bursts into an aerobic workout is a different animal entirely. After you've achieved a good level of aerobic fitness, you can begin to work higher-intensity bursts into your regimen. Increase the frequency and length of these bursts over time, and your body will adapt to them.

For example, on a day when you're outside walking, increase your walking pace for 30 seconds and then resume your normal walking pace. After doing this for a few sessions, increase to two 30-second higher-intensity walks during your walking session. You can do the same thing while biking; incorporate one to two 30-second bursts of higher-intensity pedaling during your biking session.

✔ **During the week, do different types of exercise and include rest days.** When making an exercise program for yourself, think of the rules of three: one day meditative or aerobic work, the next day resistance training, and the next day off. Allowing yourself every third day off gives your muscles time to heal and gives your body time to recharge.

You may find that you need more time off in the beginning. Maybe you need a day off after every workout. If you need it, take it, and don't feel guilty about it.

Preparing Your Body Nutritionally for Exercise

In this section, you discover specific ways to prepare your body nutritionally to get the most from your workouts. As a bonus, you'll likely minimize the exercise-induced fatigue that many people with adrenal fatigue experience.

Timing meals and workouts

Ideally, you should plan your workout between breakfast and lunch or between lunch and dinner. I (coauthor Rich) wouldn't recommend exercising first thing in the morning. Many people skimp on sleep in order to exercise before going to work, and adrenal fatigue can be associated with significant sleep-related problems. I don't want you cutting your sleep time short, and I don't want you to miss putting some nutrition in your body a couple of hours before exercising. Very late in the day after dinner is often a bad time for someone with adrenal fatigue to exercise, too, because he or she may be fatigued from the day.

If you're going to work out in the morning, be sure to start your day with foods high in protein; seeds, nuts, and avocados are great not only before but also after a workout. Juicing in the morning or taking a greens protein powder can provide your body with all the fuel it needs before a workout.

Looking at leucine

One effect of longstanding cortisol secretion is *muscle atrophy,* in which muscles have little texture or strength. On a cellular level, the muscle fibers are wasted; this condition is called *sarcopenia.*

Trying to exercise with a muscle that's wasted is about as effective as trying to drive a car when it's out of gas: You can't. You need to provide the right kind of nutrients to that muscle so it can build back up, allowing you to get the full benefits of exercise. This is where leucine comes in.

Leucine is the one amino acid that can help reverse muscle atrophy. Adrenal fatigue causes muscle *catabolism,* or breakdown; a supplement that contains leucine can help build the muscle back up.

Look for a powder that combines leucine and other amino acids, omega-3 fatty acids, and plant-based antioxidants, including chlorophyll and spirulina. I (coauthor Rich) take half of a scoop in the morning and another half scoop (a heaping tablespoon) about an hour before I exercise. I feel better, and

I think I recover a lot better after my workouts. Talk with your healthcare provider before starting this supplement. You can find many brands of these at your local health food store.

Why can't you just take leucine alone? Because when you take in amino acids, you need to take *all* of them together for nutritional and metabolic balance.

Promoting efficient energy use

In many ways, adrenal fatigue creates an energy crisis for muscle cells, so you need to account for that before exercising. Taking supplements can boost energy production by the cells, especially the muscle cells. Here's a typical pre-exercise cocktail that I recommend, especially if you're doing heavy aerobic work or muscle resistance training (remember to talk with your healthcare provider before using these supplements):

1. **Take ubiquinone (coenzyme Q_{10}) and pyrroloquinoline quinone (PQQ) with the meal prior to your workout.**

   For example, if you're planning to exercise at noon, take these supplements with your breakfast.

2. **Drink 1 to 2 glasses of alkaline water and take 2,500 to 5,000 milligrams of D-ribose powder 1 hour prior to exercise.**

   The mineralized water helps bathe the cells and eliminate any toxic buildup. You can put the D-ribose powder in the alkaline water. The water may be sweet because of the D-ribose.

You can read more about supplements and alkaline water in Chapter 11.

Avoiding certain supplements and foods

Just as knowing which supplements to take before your workouts is important, you also need to know which supplements and food to *avoid*. In particular, if you're doing muscle resistance training, your goal should be to build strength and endurance, not large muscle mass. So here are a few supplements and foods you should stay away from:

- ✔ **Creatine:** Creatine is a raw fuel for muscle, used by many power lifters and body builders to increase muscle mass. You don't need it, so you shouldn't be taking it. Creatine is a lot for your body to process. It can stress out your adrenals and kidneys.

- ✔ **High-protein-load supplements:** Although your body needs protein to function, you don't need megadoses of it. Your body and adrenal glands have to work hard to process protein. You can give your body all the protein you want, but if your muscles are in a catabolic state (experiencing muscle atrophy, as described in the earlier section "Looking at leucine"), all the protein in the world won't help. The protein powders we mention in this book aren't high in protein, and I (coauthor Rich) often use *less* than the so-called minimum amount.

✔ **Ephedra:** Ephedra is an herb that provides energy but normally with only short-term gains. It can cause dehydration and increases the risk of developing kidney stones. There are reports of serious side effects and ephedra-related deaths, and even the National Center for Complementary and Alternative Medicine has a consumer advisory about it.

✔ **Sugary foods and drinks:** I see people drinking a sugary cola drink or eating a candy bar before working out to provide them with "energy," but that's a dumb idea. You may obtain a short-term energy rise, but you put yourself at risk of bottoming out. The sugary food or drink acutely increases the workload of the adrenal glands to pump out those stress hormones, and chronic ingestion of sugary foods and drinks forces the adrenal glands to work harder. Sugar also increases inflammation, which worsens adrenal stress. Stay away from sugar before working out.

Working Out the Body Kinks

Many people — despite their best intentions and proper preparation (both physical and nutritional) — experience some soreness and muscle fatigue after their workouts. "Some" is a very gentle term; soreness may be severe. In this section, you read about two ways to work out those body kinks. The two topics in this section are also beneficial therapies in general.

Pointing out acupuncture

Acupuncture has been used for centuries. (In China, it may go back to Neolithic times, about 8500 BCE). Yes, this is the therapy where the provider sticks thin little needles in you. I (coauthor Rich) describe acupuncture to people by explaining that the body contains many energy pathways *(meridians)*; this is how your energy *(qi)* flows throughout your body. Along the pathways are many pressure points that can be accessed to bring energy and healing to afflicted areas.

Acupuncture is great for muscle, joint, and nerve pain. I've also found it beneficial in treating adrenal fatigue by reducing pain and inflammation and improving muscle flexibility and range of motion.

You want to go to someone who is a trained practitioner in acupuncture. In most states in the United States, acupuncturists are licensed (you'll likely see the abbreviation L.Ac. after the acupuncturist's name). You can go to www.nccaom.org, the website of the National Certification Commission for Acupuncture and Oriental Medicine, to find a licensed acupuncturist near you.

Some people are hesitant to use acupuncture because of the needles. Honest, the needles aren't a big deal (in fact, they're as thin as a hair), but if you want to avoid needles, *acupressure* engages those same pressure points without them. Some acupuncturists perform acupressure, but not all do. You can also look to www.nccam.org to find a practitioner of acupressure (when searching for a practitioner, check the box next to "Asian Bodywork Therapy"). Word of mouth is also a great way to find a good practitioner near you. Don't forget to ask your holistic health practitioner, who will likely be aware of good practitioners as well.

Incorporating reflexology

Your feet are much more than the two appendages you place your shoes on. Think of the soles of the feet as the place where the energy pathways of many areas of the body come together. The foot is a mini map that can provide a trained practitioner of reflexology with a snapshot of the health of the organs of your body. Each area of the foot represents a specific zone of a particular organ's energy pathway.

When the reflexology therapist presses on certain areas of your feet *(zones)*, he or she taps into a particular organ pathway and helps optimize its function (or correct a *dysfunction*). I (coauthor Rich) think reflexology therapy is invaluable not only after a workout but also for adrenal fatigue in general. It can boost organ functioning, including the adrenal glands. There's some evidence that therapists have been doing reflexology since Egypt's Sixth Dynasty (about 2450 BCE).

This form of therapy is performed by trained reflexologists, who are generally licensed by states or cities as massage therapists or "somatic practitioners." To find a licensed reflexologist near you, visit www.arcb.net/cms (the site of the American Reflexology Certification Board) and click on "Referral to a National Certificant."

You can also do some reflexology techniques at home. For details, check out *Acupressure and Reflexology For Dummies,* by Synthia Andrews and Bobbi Dempsey (Wiley).

Choosing Food: It's More Than "Don't Eat This, Don't Eat That!"

While it's essential to move, it's equally essential to fuel that movement, whether you're planning a workout or just going through your day. That goes double if you have adrenal fatigue. Here are some simple guidelines that put you in control of your food choices:

✔ **Focus on what you can eat.** It's easy to get caught up in a what-not-to-eat mode of thinking, but first focus on foods you should be eating more of; then weed out the rest over time.

Make a rainbow on your plate, with three to five servings of vegetables and fruits at every meal and pair them with your favorite protein foods to create satiety (satisfaction of your hunger).

✔ **Choose foods in their purest forms.** Whole foods give you true flavors, unlike overprocessed and excessively refined foods that add in flavoring, additives, and coloring. Processed "food" doesn't really taste good, and it further complicates identifying your food sensitivities (see Chapter 8).

✔ **Prepare your own food.** Meals don't have to be complicated to be nourishing and make your taste buds happy. Can't cook? Start with the basics: Cook a cup of rice, grill up vegetables and meats, and — ta-da! — you have a meal in under 25 minutes! The answer is yes, you *can* cook. No one is asking you to turn into Julia Child or Emeril Lagasse. Slice up an avocado, hard-boil an egg, crunch on fresh almonds, chomp on an apple, and you can build a meal.

Seeking a splash of color or more intense flavor? Look to fresh herbs (parsley, oregano, rosemary, cilantro, chives, and thyme) and spices (cumin, coriander, cinnamon, ginger, turmeric, chilies, and garlic) to take your simple dish up a notch on the flavor scale. Chapters 13 through 17 are guides to help you challenge the norm, heal you internally, and make your palette recognize the amazing flavors of foods that also heal.

✔ **Take time to enjoy your food choices.** You can't enjoy a meal if you're distracted or rushed. Give yourself time to tune in to your food. Pace yourself at the plate and focus on the flavors. Check out Chapter 17 for tips on how to really enjoy each bite.

Embrace food as your ally in your healing journey. Hippocrates said it best: "Let food be thy medicine and medicine be thy food."

Chapter 13

Managing Adrenal Fatigue on the Work Front

....

....

A major component of adrenal fatigue is stress, and one of the most common places people experience a significant amount of stress is the workplace. For many people, work-related stress can be overwhelming. In this chapter, you read about ways to reduce stress and manage your adrenal fatigue at work.

Enjoying Time Off from Work

Reasons for job dissatisfaction are many, and they can include spending an inordinate amount of time at work, feeling alienated, dealing with hypercritical and unfriendly coworkers and bosses, and feeling a lack of ownership and motivation for the job you're paid to do. You may have anxiety about being laid off or forced into early retirement. In addition, jobs are scarce, and you may feel that you're lucky to have a job.

If any of these situations apply to you, you're probably stressed by your job, so enjoying time off from work may be just what the doctor ordered for your adrenal fatigue. In this section, you read about options for taking time off, ranging from taking vacations to flat-out quitting your job. But first, you need to recognize symptoms of burnout.

Before making any major work-related decisions, know where you stand and what your goals are. Do you spend a lot? Is your goal to have the big house and fancy car? Or would you be happier with a smaller house, a used car, and more free time? By understanding who you are — and what you need versus what you want — you're able to make better-informed decisions.

Recognizing the need to take time off

Burnout is the term psychologists use to describe diminished interest in work. You could quit your job, but for most people, that's not an option. You have rent or mortgages to pay, a family that depends on you, and your kids' college tuition to worry about.

If you're at least aware of burnout, you can recognize when you need to take some time off work to recharge your batteries. Here are some common signs:

- You're developing a short fuse and find yourself snapping at everyone and everything.

- You feel completely unmotivated to go to work.

- You've become very critical of others.

- Your eating habits have changed. Maybe you find yourself eating more, or maybe you've completely lost your appetite.

- You're drinking or using drugs to help you get through your workday.

If one or more of these symptoms describes the changes you've undergone, you may have burnout, which can lead to or worsen adrenal fatigue.

So what causes burnout? One of the biggest misconceptions concerning burnout is that it depends on the number of hours you spend at work. Although that's a significant contributing factor, it isn't the whole story. Factors that you haven't even thought about may be at play. They can include

- **Work-family dysfunction:** You may spend more time with your work family than with your regular family. That means you're putting up with personalities, values, and behaviors that may not match yours.

- **Lack of socialization:** Maybe you sit in a cubicle all day and don't interact with another human being during your whole shift. But humans are social animals. People need some degree of social interaction, feedback on work performance, and planning and expectations concerning the job itself.

- **Lack of autonomy and empowerment:** Studies show that workers feel empowered when they have some say and have some flexibility to have that say about the final product (or at least the process). It's not just about money; in fact, money issues are just one factor among many concerning dissatisfaction in the workplace. What can be depressing is the feeling that you don't matter and that no one cares what you think.

Burnout is actually a classified syndrome. The earlier you recognize the symptoms, the better your chances of getting better. The advanced stages of burnout syndrome may require more intervention than simply taking time off work, because those stages can include clinical depression and thoughts of suicide. A holistic treatment strategy is often needed in treating burnout syndrome, and that strategy can include *cognitive behavior therapy.* This type of therapy is geared toward changing how you think about yourself and the world around you. It focuses on thought patterns as well as internal and external influences that can affect your thought patterns.

Making sure you don't waste your vacation days

When was the last time you took a vacation? If you have to think for more than a few seconds, then you definitely need to take one — and pronto!

Countering excuses not to go

Of course, people are full of excuses as to why they don't take vacations. Here are some:

- ✔ **"This department couldn't run without me."** With all due respect for your skills, it can. Go on vacation.

- ✔ **"It's too expensive to travel somewhere."** With the right planning, you can travel very inexpensively. With travel websites such as www. priceline.com and www.hotwire.com, you can look for the best deals. You'll have fun and save a lot of money at the same time.

Taking a vacation doesn't mean you have to go anywhere. Don't forget the *staycation,* where you do leisure activities within driving distance of your home and sleep in your own bed at night. The idea of a vacation is to relax. Relaxation occurs in the mind first and foremost. For some people, just being at home and away from work is a vacation.

- ✔ **"I'm waiting until retirement."** This is one excuse that you really need to rethink. First, you may die or become disabled before retirement. Take the vacation now. Second, many people choose to delay their retirement, often waiting years. Here's an irony: The need for health insurance is a major reason to continue working, so you get sicker working to maintain health insurance for when you're sick. Go figure.

If you can, consider making vacations *mini-retirements.* Why wait until retirement to do things you want to do right now, especially in unpredictable economic times? The important thing is to space out your vacation days throughout the year so that you don't spend all your vacation time too early, leaving you unable to take a proper vacation break later on.

Enjoying your time off

Give yourself permission to do whatever you consider to be fun on your vacation. Maybe you just want to walk around a big city. Maybe you're more adventurous and you want to explore a foreign country or go to the mountains. Maybe you just want to spend a day by the beach. The important thing is that you give yourself permission to relax, have fun, and enjoy!

Consider taking a cruise. Being on a cruise has a lot of advantages. Your trip is already planned, your lodgings and food are taken care of (the cost of taking a cruise can be a lot less than staying at a hotel and paying for meals), you don't need to worry about the travel (hopefully the ship is sound), you get to meet a lot of new people, and you see places you likely haven't seen before. The cruise can also promote great quality time with the family.

If you're single, there's nothing better than a singles cruise, especially if you want to meet someone. Being single also means that you're free to see the world. Why not consider a backpacking trip through Europe?

Wherever you go — or even if you stay home — here are a couple of ways to help you relax and make sure your vacation stays stress-free:

- **Don't forget the power of visualization!** A few days before beginning your time off, visualize yourself having a relaxing moment, whether that means sitting on a beach or spending quality time with your family.

- **Avoid work-related technology as much as possible.** Turn off the cellphone, shut off the beeper, unplug the computer. Stay away from the iPod, and just focus on relaxing!

Switching the amount or location of the work you do

Today's worker has more schedule and location options than ever before. Many employers are looking for ways to decrease costs and increase employee satisfaction. Decreasing to part-time work (if you're able), working at home (WAH), and contracting are options. For some people, decreasing the time spent working and/or changing the scenery may be just the ticket to curing burnout.

The pleasure of part time

Sometimes part-time jobs are advertised. In other cases, you need to suggest to your boss that if you go from full time to part time, you'll increase your overall productivity. The change may also increase your happiness and job satisfaction. Other advantages to part-time work include the following:

✔ It can offer more flexibility, depending on the nature of job.

✔ You can devote more time to friends and spend meaningful quality time with family.

✔ You get some "me" time. This includes time for relaxation, exercise, sleep, and proper nutrition.

The most obvious casualty of changing to part-time work is your company-paid health insurance: You'll lose it. However, some companies don't offer health insurance anyway, so you're not losing a thing. In fact, with the Affordable Care Act in the United States, you may be able to find good health insurance partially subsidized by the government.

Working at home: Hurrah for WAH

Working at home can not only increase your overall productivity but also increase your happiness and job satisfaction. You may be able to accomplish the same amount of work you normally do but in a lot less time because your work environment (your home) is much more pleasant. Being able to work at home offers several advantages:

✔ It eliminates travel time and the stress of the morning and evening commutes.

✔ It saves you a lot of money, including gas, parking, and car maintenance costs.

✔ It allows you to have breakfast with your family and see your kids off to school in the morning. If you work at home, you're there when your kids come home from school, and you can have dinner with your family. For many, the ability to have this kind of quality family time is priceless.

Some employers don't trust you to work at home, but others actually encourage telecommuting, at least for part of the week.

Working at home is not without its challenges. One of the biggest hurdles that many people face when beginning to work at home is finding "work time." Kids, family, and other commitments can eat into your day. It's important to establish hours during the day that are yours and yours only so you can get your work done. Some people may miss the socialization at the office, but with technology, including Skype and e-mail, this is less of an issue.

The appeal of contracting

Contractors (sometimes called "consultants") work through a temp agency. Contract jobs often last about 3 months, and the money is better than working as a captive employee. Because employers are trying to pinch pennies, the number of contract jobs in the United States is increasing. You can take

Changing where you work

For some people, although they like their jobs, the physical location causes increased stress and anger. A cubicle may not be the most productive place for you to work. Maybe you can change your workspace. See whether you can physically work somewhere else in the building. For example, can you work out of the company library for one day per week? Or what about working from the bookstore across the street? Or working outdoors a few hours each day? Progressive companies are searching for ways to maximize not only the productivity but also the job satisfaction of each employee.

In some cases, the cause of stress is the branch office where you work. Maybe you can transfer to another facility. Such a transition can offer a fresh beginning, a new opportunity. On the other hand, going to a new location, especially if you're moving far away from relatives and friends, can be very stressful for you and your family. Before making any major decision concerning a work change, be sure that you've thoroughly reviewed the risks and benefits.

as much time between contracts as you like. No, there's no health insurance, but you can buy private health insurance. You never have to stress about losing your job unexpectedly, because the day you start a contract, you know it's going to end. Some people use a temp agency for finding a new job; others may find contract-based jobs on their own.

Networking is so important when you're thinking about moving on to another position. Every person that you meet is an opportunity to establish a potential contact.

Changing your job

Sometimes, you have no choice but to change jobs if you want to reduce stress. For many people, changing jobs is a last resort, and it can be scary — especially if you've been in one position or at one company for a long time. But for others, the change is invigorating. You get an opportunity to pursue things that you may have been hesitant to do before.

Granted, the stress of a job search can be big. You write a lot of resumes and have to use your network of friends. But if you can pull it off, a job change may pay off in a big way.

If you've quit your job, been laid off, or are contemplating a career change, the services of a career coach can be invaluable. Career coaches can help you clarify your thoughts, find out what you really want to do, and figure out how to get there. They can help you think of career options that you may not have thought of on your own. Don't be afraid to ask for help, because it could be the best thing you can do to change careers or revive your career. Where can you find a reputable career coach? An excellent resource is the National Career Development Association (www.ncda.org).

Taking Time Out during the Workday

Taking a timeout during the workday is something you can and should consider to relieve stress and ease your adrenal fatigue. Many of the items in this section take little or no time at all. You just need to actively plan and be committed to taking the time.

Time management is vital not only for making you more efficient and productive at work but also for building in breaks and "me" time. A good resource for planning your day is *Successful Time Management For Dummies,* by Dirk Zeller (Wiley).

Turning off technology and talking face-to-face

Although electronic communication and social media have revolutionized how people communicate, in some ways it has dramatically cut down on *meaningful* person-to-person interaction. E-mails, faxes, memos, and text messaging can be efficient, but they're impersonal and often aren't as effective as real, personal contact.

Twitter tweets and Facebook posts combine to produce information overload, especially first thing in the morning. That overload can be extremely stressful. Going to work only to sit down and open up pages of tweets and posts (and e-mails, too!) that need review and response can be a cause of mega-stress.

Consider taking a technology timeout. Set aside a time where you step away from anything electronic — that means stepping away from your computer and turning off your cellphone and any other electronic device you have. Break the cycle by getting out of your cubicle and having real conversations with live people. (If you work at a bank or in retail, personal interactions are easier.) Walk around and say hello. See how you can foster a friendlier work atmosphere simply by making communication more personal.

Meditating for a few minutes

Meditation is a process that can take as little as a few minutes. The purpose of meditation is to center yourself. With the day-to-day goings-on at work, you can become scattered and unfocused. Believe us — "centered" is better than "scattered."

At the bare minimum, perform breathing exercises (see Chapter 6) sitting in your office chair a few times throughout the day. Fear and panic will go away, and you'll have a less stressful workday. If you want something more, please refer to Chapter 12 for info on yoga and t'ai chi.

Using your senses to relax

Most people were born with five senses (and we think some folks have some form of a sixth sense as well). You can use your senses at work (and at home, too) not only to cope with stress but also to promote overall health. Ways to relax with your senses include the following:

✔ **Music therapy:** Listening to soothing and relaxing music during your workday can have a very relaxing effect. Research shows that music therapy can reduce stress, promote relaxation, and even reduce pain.

✔ **Aromatherapy:** The scent of lavender oil at your desk at work can have a relaxing effect and reduce stress levels.

✔ **Visual observation:** Visual observation opens up worlds to you. If you arrive at work early in the day or leave late, watch the sunrise or sunset. At lunch, lie down on a lawn (if there's one nearby) and watch what goes on in the grass (you may see bugs, flowers, and marvelous growth patterns). Consider taking a 2-hour lunch and dashing to a local art museum or gallery.

Don't forget to include your sense of sight in the office! If you're spending 8 hours a day staring at a computer, doesn't it pay to look at something relaxing on your screen? Consider choosing a soothing scene as your screen's wallpaper. If you're able, add plants and some nature pictures to your office or cubicle.

Making the most of your lunch hour

Many people just spend the lunch hour trying to catch up on the day's work. They often forget that they even have a lunch hour. Bad idea. Realize that your lunch hour should be a transition point from the morning to the afternoon. You need to claim that time for yourself. It should be a time for rest, relaxation, and rejuvenation.

Take some time for meditation during your lunch hour. The noon lunch hour can be an invaluable time for getting in some exercise, too — see the next section for details.

Building Exercise into Your Workday

Exercise is beneficial for adrenal fatigue patients because it relieves stress, helps build endurance and strength, and can make you feel better all around. One of the most common complaints we hear is that people don't have time to work out. They work all day and they're too tired to exercise at home. One option is to build exercise into and around your workday.

Going places

One of the easiest ways to work exercise into your day is to forgo the elevator and other machines that get you from here to there.

Bicycling or walking to and from work

How do you get to work in the morning? Maybe you drive, take a bus, or take the train. If your work is close, consider bicycling to work. If you live in the city, where there's heavy traffic, you may actually get to work faster than you would driving a car. If you take a bus or train, consider getting off at an earlier stop and walking to work. ***Note:*** Don't forget to put on your sneakers before walking to or from work. Using proper footwear is important, especially if you're going to embark on a walking program.

Taking the stairs

When you're at work, avoid using the elevator and take the stairs instead. An average sized person can burn about 8 calories walking up a flight of stairs. Contrast this to taking an elevator, in which you burn only about 2 calories (maybe 3 if you pace back and forth in the elevator!).

What goes up must come down! You actually burn a similar number of calories walking down the stairs as you do walking up. You also increase your body's metabolism, which means that throughout the course of the day, you burn calories more efficiently.

Moving during the day

Your body was made for movement. Any movement that you can get is going to be positively beneficial. In this section, you read about ways you can increase your fitness level while at work.

Working your glutes and quads

If you were to ask an average person how many times he or she uses the bathroom each day, the answer would probably be six to eight times. If you were to ask how often he or she exercises during those times, the answer would likely be none.

Get some exercise by using the bathroom. How? Simply avoid sitting on the toilet seat. Squatting not only builds up your quadriceps muscles but also strengthens your gluteus maximus muscles in the process. Think of this quality time as a way to perform isometric exercises.

Also note that while sitting at your desk, you can tighten and relax various muscle groups, so you can get exercise benefits even while you're sitting. Start holding each muscle group for a count of five, and then release. At a minimum, you should aim to do this twice for each muscle group during the workday: once in the morning and once after lunch.

Getting up and moving every hour

If your job is sitting at a desk for 8 to 10 hours a day, you should get up at least once an hour if possible. That's what research studies show. Your body was meant to move. Get up, walk around, and stretch your muscles for a few minutes.

A study in the medical journal *Diabetes Care* (published in 2011) demonstrated that the less time you spend sitting at your desk, the better your overall health. In particular, there's a decrease in waist size, decrease in body mass index (high BMI correlates with obesity), and a reduction in triglyceride levels. There's a decrease in glucose levels as well.

Walking at lunchtime

Bring a pair of sneakers to work, and you can walk at lunchtime. This is already commonplace in communities where the weather is relatively good and the corporate culture encourages it (Silicon Valley, for example). In some workplaces, you'll see many a co-worker at lunchtime walking around the parking lots or using the walkways between buildings.

Any walking is better than not walking at all. Even if all you can do is walk 15 minutes, your health will improve, your stress levels will lower, and you'll be in a better mood to start the afternoon.

Exercising on the way home from work

After a long workday (especially if you've been sitting behind a desk for 8 hours), exercising in a gym can be just what the doctor ordered. Stop on the way home and just do it. The benefits of a gym membership are many. In addition to using the free weights and machines, you can take exercise classes, including aerobics and karate. And exercising in a group can be a great motivating experience.

 Many companies are starting to recognize that a healthy and fit employee is a productive employee. Some companies arrange for reduced prices at local fitness centers to encourage their employees to use the facilities. A few have free fitness centers on campus. Check with your human resources department to find out whether your company can get you a discount.

 Some insurance plans reduce or refund part of your health insurance premiums (or don't increase them) if you maintain a consistent exercise program. The plan may require that you exercise at the gym a few times a week or walk a certain distance every day. Check your insurance plan to see whether there's a deal that applies to you.

Eating and Drinking Well during the Workday

What you put (or don't put) in your body while at work can exacerbate any stressful situation. The two biggest culprits at work are caffeinated beverages and sugar, but it's also important to eat all your meals (no skipping!) and avoid alcohol.

Eating all your meals

Missing breakfast is a no-no, and of course, the best breakfast is one you make yourself at home, because it can provide you with protein, complex carbs, and fruit. If you're constantly in a hurry in the morning before work, drinking a greens powder shake in the morning provides some antioxidant value, protein to satiate you, and servings of fruits and vegetables; it also normalizes your pH, which is so important in decreasing cellular stress. You can visit your local health food store and see the many options you have to choose from. You usually add greens powders to an 8-ounce glass of water.

Going through the drive-through isn't a great choice, especially for folks with adrenal fatigue. Those breakfasts have some pretty poor nutrition and a lot of fat and sodium. If you *must* go through the fast food drive-through, aim for the healthiest choice on the menu.

If you're so rushed in the morning that you can't eat breakfast, at least have a healthy snack in the morning. You want to be sure that you eat something.

Skipping a meal at work isn't a good idea, either — it's a terrible idea, in fact. Don't miss lunch! Your body needs the fuel that only lunch provides. Skipping lunch will make you tired, irritable, and famished by the time dinner comes, making you want to eat everything in sight. You and your adrenal glands need nutrients in the afternoon to function efficiently and effectively.

If you're able, consider eating smaller meals throughout the day. If possible, have a healthy snack in the middle of the morning, which can help keep you from gorging yourself at lunch (after which you may feel like falling asleep in the middle of the afternoon). Have an afternoon snack, too. Eating smaller meals throughout the day is easier on your body than pigging out at lunch or dinner. You can find some great snack recipes in Chapter 17.

Eating great food to keep you going

If you want to feel great and beat adrenal fatigue during your workday, then it makes sense that you need to eat great food. Your breakfast choices set the tone for the beginning of the day, and eating a nutritious lunch is key to feeling great the whole afternoon.

Have some fruit for breakfast. Consider substituting an apple for the doughnut or an orange for the bagel. Also think about having a vegetable-based meal in the morning. Salads don't just have to be for lunch and dinner! And be sure to include some protein in a morning meal. That way, you won't be starving for lunch, and you'll decrease your risk of bottoming out. You'll also better maintain your energy during the day.

Eating healthy at work means being prepared. Consider packing your own lunch to bring to work with you. Keep some healthy snack options on hand as well. When dining out with coworkers, make it a point to look for and ask the waiter about the healthy food choices on the menu. Check out some delicious recipes in Part IV.

Avoiding foods and drinks that tax your adrenals

Some foods and drinks can worsen adrenal fatigue and make you feel bloated and tired. In this section, you read about decreasing your caffeine intake and reducing your sugar intake as much as possible.

Decreasing your caffeine intake

Think about how many cups of coffee you have daily. Add to this the other caffeinated beverages, including iced tea, carbonated beverages, and energy drinks, that you consume during the day. You may be giving your heart and your adrenal glands quite a workout. Don't do it! Here are some tips for reducing your caffeine intake:

✔ **If you've been drinking mega cups of coffee a day for a long time, then reduce your intake gradually.** Start making your coffee half regular, half decaf; then, over the course of a few weeks, convert to decaffeinated coffee. Switching to smaller mugs or smaller coffee cups is also an option. Although coffee has many health benefits, the caffeine can be detrimental.

✔ **Stop going to the vending machine to get soft drinks during your breaks.** In addition to buying a carbonated soft drink during the day, many people get an unhealthy snack. Bring a caffeine-free beverage in a thermos from home if possible. Increase your water intake. Water is the only real thirst-quencher.

Great substitutes for caffeinated beverages include green tea, filtered/alkalinized water, and decaffeinated coffee. If you want a beverage that's tasty and healthy, consider bringing a juicer to the office break room.

Small cup, big effect

You almost have to take a college course to understand the various forms of caffeinated beverages that are out there — espresso, cappuccino, latte, and so on. The cups for espressos and cappuccinos are smaller than those for regular coffee, but these drinks have a strong flavor and deliver a wallop of caffeine. So don't let the size of the cups fool you — a small cup can pack quite a punch.

Substituting for sugar

What's a typical breakfast in a break room? Well, it can include doughnuts (yes, even the ones with the cream and jelly in them), muffins, and/or bagels. Trust us when we say that simple sugars and items made from white flour aren't the best thing to have in the morning.

Between the sugar rush from the doughnut and the caffeine rush from the morning java, your adrenal glands are in for a world of hurt. If this constitutes your morning routine, you're at a severe risk of crashing later in the day due to low blood sugar, especially in advanced stages of adrenal fatigue.

You should also try to minimize your intake of sugary foods during lunch and at dinner. After lunch, skip the sweet dessert that may be offered. Don't go back into the break room and take that doughnut you may have missed in the morning. Do your best to stay away from the vending machines.

If you find that you do have a sweet tooth, especially in the morning, consider using stevia, an acceptable sugar substitute. Stay away from artificial sweeteners in your coffee and other drinks if possible.

If you find that you have a persistent sugar craving, you may have a yeast overgrowth problem. Jump to Chapter 11 to find out how to eliminate yeast and restore your bowel health. A happy bowel can really help decrease sugar cravings.

Avoiding alcohol

You may think that you're relieving stress after work by drinking a cold one (or two), but you're doing yourself more harm than good. Alcohol is a depressant of the central nervous system. It increases the risk of dehydration and can cause you to become depleted of much-needed electrolytes and minerals, especially magnesium. This can lead to adrenal fatigue as well as worsen already-existing adrenal fatigue.

Drinking alcohol frequently can set you up for a chemical dependence. If you drink the night before, you may find yourself needing coffee in the morning to get you going. Then you may use alcohol in the evening to calm down. Your body becomes a mixture of chemicals to get you up in the morning and settle you down in the afternoon and evening.

Battling Brain Fog in the Workplace

If you're experiencing symptoms of brain fog at work, including memory problems, confusion, depression, and/or an inability to concentrate, you likely have adrenal fatigue. Your adrenal fatigue is likely at a moderate stage, but you still need to be further evaluated and take steps to prevent your symptoms from worsening. In the meantime, here are some things you can do to help manage brain fog at work:

- **Eat veggies, complex carbs, and protein.** If you have symptoms that suggest brain fog, avoid eating carbs, especially simple carbs like white bread and sugar, at work. They only make the symptoms worse. If anything, change your diet to include more vegetables (ones that have an alkaline bent, like broccoli and kale). In fact, you can save a buck by bringing cucumber spears and carrot sticks from home. Also be sure that you're consuming an adequate amount of protein (like chicken or fish).

  When the coffee cart or lunch truck comes around, avoid powdery doughnuts, sugary soft drinks, and other cheap thrills if you can. Skip excess caffeine and alcoholic beverages, too, because they only make brain fog worse.

- **Go outside.** Be sure you build up your store of vitamin D. It's free, because you get it just by going outside. Get some sun; 20 minutes in the middle of the day can provide enough vitamin D to prevent deficiency of this important vitamin. In the winter, you'll likely need to take a vitamin D supplement. See Chapter 11 for info on supplementation.

- **Pay attention to the eliminators.** In addition to the adrenal glands, two organs you want to pay attention to if brain fog is present are the liver and the kidneys. The liver is responsible for processing toxins, medications, and food that you eat; the kidneys are responsible for eliminating them from the body.

  Optimizing liver and kidney function is crucial. Drink mineralized water with an alkaline pH to flush the toxins out of the body and keep the kidneys in good shape. Eating foods that promote healthy intestinal flora can help decrease the workload of the liver; yogurt is a great option. For more information on supplements you can take to help treat brain fog and adrenal fatigue, see Chapter 11.

- **Normalize your morning pH.** If you're suffering from brain fog, normalizing your morning urine pH is extremely important. If a urine pH test strip shows your pH is low in the morning — below 6.5 — take an alkaline-based drink like alkaline water with a squeeze of lemon added to it. Please refer to Chapter 5 for info on measuring your pH.

Part IV
Trying Sensational Recipes to Battle Adrenal Fatigue

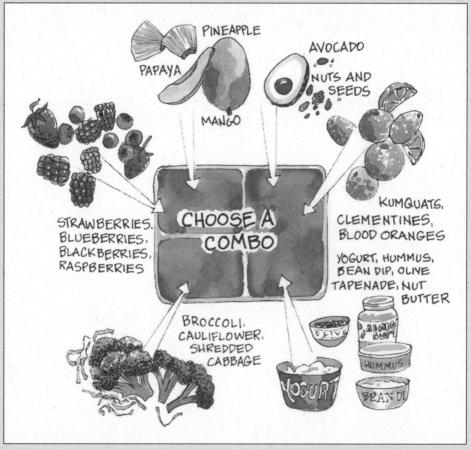

Illustration by Elizabeth Kurtzman

In this part...

- ✔ Make great breakfasts that will keep you energized throughout your morning. Identify the components of a healthy breakfast and discover some options for both juicing and solid meals.

- ✔ Discover the secrets to preparing tasty, nutritious lunches. Find guidance on boosting your protein intake and packing on-the-go lunches.

- ✔ Whip up delicious, healthy, satisfying dinners that are packed with antioxidants and healing nutrients.

- ✔ Pick up the key to fun living though healthy, nutritious desserts and snacks. Satisfy your cravings with something salty or sweet and learn how to enjoy each bite.

Chapter 14

Beginning with Energizing Breakfasts

In This Chapter

▶ Exploring the basics of breakfast

▶ Kicking off your day with simple vegetable and fruit juices

▶ Incorporating protein and whole grains

Skipping breakfast alters your metabolism and can be a recipe for disaster. Come lunch hour, you'll likely feel fatigued and famished, which can lead to overeating at lunch. Then, consuming more food than you need to at one sitting can make you sleepy and lethargic during the afternoon. If your adrenal system is already stressed, then these poor eating habits can lead to adrenal exhaustion.

Eating breakfast is important for everyone, especially adrenal fatigue patients. Seriously, don't skip breakfast! Breakfast gives you the energy you need to greet the day. In this chapter, we talk about the components of a healthy breakfast and describe some options for both homemade juice blends and solid meals. We wrap up with a number of delicious breakfast recipes for you to try. *Note:* Recipes listed with a tomato icon are vegetarian.

Examining Breakfast Essentials

What are the components of a successful, high-quality morning program to begin your day? Here are some essentials:

▸ **Choose complex-carbohydrate foods over simple-carbohydrate foods.** The least-processed foods are always the best. Look for whole-grain foods with more than 3 grams of fiber per serving. Refer to Chapter 7 for reasons you may want to choose grains other than wheat, rye, and barley, which contain gluten.

✔ **Include foods higher in protein.** Foods with at least 5 grams of protein per ounce are best. You can also combine vegetarian sources to achieve higher protein amounts in a meal.

✔ **Add vegetables, whether by juicing or simply snacking.** Vegetables give you a boost of vitamins, minerals, and fiber.

✔ **Forage for fats from nuts and avocados to help hold you over until your next meal.** Nuts and avocados are especially good for adrenal fatigue patients because of their essential fats.

✔ **Eat small portions to help keep you from feeling groggy after the meal.** Need a portion guide? Pull out your dessert plates and use them to guide you to a healthy portion.

In addition to eating breakfast, you can start your day by meditating and writing a list of things for which you're grateful. A gratitude list lets you kick-start your day on a positive note instead of feeling rushed and adding stress to an already stressed body.

Organic or not organic? That's everyone's question!

Before you add more stress to your plate by piling on the notion that a green is good for you only if it's organic, stop. First, focus on taking in more fruits and vegetables. This is the key concern: Get in more of the essential nutrients, phytochemicals, and antioxidants that fresh produce boasts. Next, look to the Dirty Dozen and the Clean Fifteen as guides on which foods to buy organic. The Environmental Working Group (EWG) puts out its lists every year, as practices and products change. Check www. ewg.org for its most up-to-date lists.

In 2013, the following made the Dirty Dozen Plus list. Grab for these foods first in the organic bin:

✔ Apples

✔ Celery

✔ Cherry tomatoes

✔ Cucumbers

✔ Grapes

✔ Hot peppers

✔ Imported nectarines

✔ Peaches

✔ Potatoes

✔ Spinach

✔ Strawberries

✔ Sweet bell peppers

✔ Kale and collard greens

✔ Summer squash

The Clean Fifteen for 2013 includes asparagus, avocados, cabbage, cantaloupe, sweet corn, eggplant, grapefruit, kiwis, mangos, mushrooms, onions, papayas, pineapples, frozen sweet peas, and sweet potatoes. You can skip organic versions of these foods, knowing that these produce items are cleaner than the rest.

Juicing It Up

Vegetables and fruits are your best choices for maximum nutrient density. In addition to being loaded with vitamins and minerals, vegetables and fruits pack a potent antioxidant punch. Most Americans eat only two to three servings per day, whereas the American Cancer Society recommends consuming five to nine servings per day. Packing in fresh fruits and vegetables is essential for optimal health, so aim for the higher end of the recommended range.

Vegetable and fruit juicing may be the solution for boosting your intake. A 6-ounce serving of juice is equivalent to one vegetable or fruit serving. You don't have to become a juicing fanatic or start on an all-juice fast, but juicing is a great way to get a greater variety and quantity of vegetables into your diet.

Note that juicing removes most fiber from vegetables and fruits, so if your diet needs more fiber, consider blending in place of juicing. We include a great smoothie recipe in Chapter 17. Great options for a high-powered blender are the Vitamix, Blendtec, or Ninja.

Start juicing familiar fruits and vegetables and then work your way to more unique combinations. Sweeter vegetables, such as carrots, are an easy starting point. Fruits can mask vegetable flavors and deliver plenty of antioxidants. The rule of thumb is to have a greater quantity of vegetables than fruit in your juice or smoothie to keep the calorie content lower. (You can find some great juice blends in the later sidebar "Juicing combinations.")

When buying a juicer, look for the following attributes:

- ✔ Simple to clean
- ✔ Easy to use
- ✔ Able to extract juice from leafy vegetables and wheat grass
- ✔ Motor warranty greater than 5 years

Two main types of juicers are available — centrifugal juicers and masticating juicers — and they operate very differently from one another.

Centrifugal juicers

Centrifugal juicers are the more common type, and their lower cost makes them appealing to consumers. A plate inside a centrifugal juicer grates the fruit or vegetable into very small pieces, and the juice is strained out through a mesh basket that spins extremely fast (6,500–13,500 rpm). These juicers work very much like the spin cycle in your washing machine as they separate juice from pulp.

Juicing combinations

For a tasty way to sip your nutrients, use your juicer to extract juice from one of the following combinations of ingredients. Stir the juice and store it in a glass jar. Each of these combinations should provide 18 ounces of juice, giving you three 6-ounce servings for your day. Juices are best when consumed within 24 hours of preparation. **Note:** If you're concerned with the sugar content of these juices, please note that only 6 ounces are recommended at one time. Look for information on the glycemic index in Chapter 17.

Beeting Stress

- 2 small beets
- 1 inch gingerroot
- 4 medium oranges, peeled
- 1 small green apple, cored

Enzymatic Bliss

- 1 cup peeled papaya
- 1 cup peeled pineapple
- 1 cup peeled mango
- 2 medium celery stalks
- 1 medium cucumber

Vary It! This is a great recipe for blending as well as juicing! Blend your fresh fruits to a smooth consistency while you juice your vegetables; then blend the vegetable juice into your creamy fruit pulp.

Going Green

- 1 medium cucumber
- 4 large kale leaves

- 1 cup peeled pineapple
- ¼ of a jalapeño (if you desire less heat, be sure to remove the seeds)
- 1 small green apple, cored

Loving Your Liver

- 2 fennel bulbs and stalks
- 2 small green apples, cored
- 1 medium lemon, peeled

Savory Red

- 6 medium celery stalks
- 6 medium tomatoes
- 1 medium cucumber
- 1 garlic clove
- 4 medium carrots, peeled
- 1 tablespoon fresh oregano
- 1 medium lime, peeled

Turning Orange

- ½ inch fresh turmeric
- 8 medium carrots, peeled
- 1 inch gingerroot
- 3 medium oranges, peeled

Tip: You can store fresh turmeric in the freezer for later use. Be sure to defrost before juicing. If your juicer turns a little orange, simply wipe it down with a paper towel dipped in olive or coconut oil.

Centrifugal juicers have three main drawbacks:

- ✔ They can be loud due to the spinning motor inside the machine.

- ✔ Because these machines operate very fast, the ingredients are prone to oxidation due to the heat produced, so your juice may not last as long if you're planning on saving it for later.

- ✔ They lack efficiency in juicing leafy greens, so you may end up having to buy more produce in the long run.

You can find a centrifugal juicer for under $100; however, read the reviews before making a purchase.

Masticating juicers

Masticating juicers slowly grind the ingredients, almost mimicking how humans chew food — hence the name "masticating." These juicers grind ingredients very slowly (about 80 rpm), and this slow speed decreases oxidation, which lets your juice keep longer (48 to 72 hours). Masticating juicers excel at juicing leafy greens and are very popular for juicing wheatgrass.

Masticating juicers have two main drawbacks:

- ✔ First is price — some of these machines have a starting cost of $250 to $300.

- ✔ Second is the number of parts used to operate the machine. You may need to spend a little bit more time each morning over the kitchen sink making sure your machine is clean for the next juicing session.

Making a Solid Start to Your Day

Although juicing is a great way to start your day (see the preceding section), you may want to add solid foods as well. Research shows that solid foods increase *satiety* (the condition of feeling comfortable after consuming food), so if you want to feel full, be sure to combine a serving of vegetable juice with something solid at breakfast. The following sections discuss two types of solid food to consider: those containing protein and those containing whole grains.

Processing protein

Protein is a critical component of breakfast. Research shows that consuming 30 grams of protein at each meal influences the expression of hormones related to feeling full and increases the psychological sense of satiety. Two particular hormones influenced by protein at each meal are leptin and ghrelin. *Leptin* signals fullness to the brain, and *ghrelin* initiates hunger or readiness to eat.

Researchers are continually studying leptin and ghrelin in relation to obesity. They've found that tuning in to whether you're hungry or full is key. You want to recognize foods that help you feel satiated so you won't want to overconsume. That's what will get you to a desirable weight.

Adding whole grains

Whole grains have long been touted for their fiber, antioxidant, vitamin, and mineral content. In the following recipes, we step away from typical gluten-based products and move toward whole grains and seeds such as quinoa and millet. (We cover the ill effects of gluten on intestinal health in Chapter 7.)

Gluten is a protein consisting of glutenin and gliadin. If you want to avoid gluten, here's a quick list of common offenders: wheat, barley, rye, triticale, bulgur, farina, semolina, and beer. Some people have a true wheat allergy, whereas others are sensitive to gluten. Have a physician test you for gluten intolerance prior to eliminating gluten from your diet, or you may get false results.

Fixing fast breakfasts

If your schedule is tight in the morning and you feel too rushed to sit down to breakfast, opt for one of these simple on-the-go breakfast ideas. They're a mixture of protein and carbohydrates.

- 8 ounces Greek yogurt, 1 cup berries, and ¼ cup granola

- 1 slice sprouted grain toast, ¼ cup hummus, ¼ cup sprouts, and 1 boiled egg

- 2 boiled eggs, 6 whole-grain gluten-free crackers, and 6 ounces vegetable juice

- ¼ cup black beans, 3 ounces lean beef, and 2 tablespoons salsa on a warm corn tortilla

- Chocolate, Banana, and Almond Butter Smoothie; see the recipe in Chapter 17

Breakfast Quinoa

Prep time: 2 min • **Cook time:** 25 min • **Yield:** 4 servings

Ingredients	Directions
2 cups unsweetened, boxed or refrigerated coconut milk (not canned), plus more for serving	*1* In a 2-quart saucepan, bring the coconut milk to a boil over medium-high heat.
1 cup quinoa, rinsed	*2* Add the quinoa to the saucepan and return the mixture to a boil, stirring constantly. Reduce the heat to low and simmer, covered, until three-quarters of the milk has been absorbed, about 15 minutes.
3 tablespoons maple syrup, plus more for serving	
⅛ teaspoon ground cinnamon, plus more for serving	*3* Stir in the maple syrup and cinnamon. Cook, covered, until almost all the milk has been absorbed, about 8 minutes.
1 cup fresh blueberries, plus more for serving	
	4 Remove the saucepan from the heat and stir in the blueberries.
	5 Divide the quinoa among four bowls and serve with additional milk, maple syrup, cinnamon, and blueberries.

Per serving: Calories 263 (From Fat 53); Fat 6g (Saturated 2g); Cholesterol 0mg; Sodium 20mg; Carbohydrate 46g (Dietary Fiber 12g); Protein 7g.

Vary It! Feel free to replace the coconut milk with almond milk. You can also add different fruits such as bananas to change the flavor.

Note: This dish reheats well. Just add a splash of coconut milk and you can zap it in the microwave.

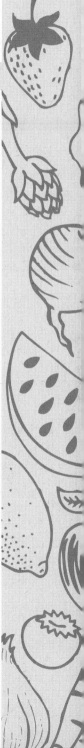

Tart Cherry Muesli

Prep time: 1 min • **Yield:** 12 servings (½ cup each)

Ingredients	Directions
1 cup dried tart cherries (no sugar added)	**1** In a large bowl, mix together the cherries, blueberries, oats, puffed millet, walnuts, seeds, and cinnamon. Store the mix in an airtight container for up to 1 month.
½ cup dried blueberries	
2 cups gluten-free oats	
1 cup puffed millet cereal	
1 cup walnuts, chopped	
½ cup pumpkin or sunflower seeds	
Cinnamon to taste (optional)	

Per serving: Calories 275 (From Fat 100); Fat 11g (Saturated 0g); Cholesterol 0mg; Sodium 1mg; Carbohydrate 37g (Dietary Fiber 8g); Protein 9g.

Note: Millet isn't just for the birds! This nutrient-dense grain is alkaline and gluten-free. Mild in flavor and fluffy in texture, millet cooks up like rice but provides a nutty taste.

Vary It! After you prepare muesli, you can add warm coconut or almond milk, chilled Greek yogurt, or kefir for serving. Tart Cherry Muesli is also a great addition to Açaí Bowls (see the next recipe).

There's something sweet about tart cherries

Tart cherries contain melatonin, which is the hormone that helps people fall asleep. Tart cherries also contain antioxidants, mainly anthocyanins, which gives cherries their bright red color. These phytochemicals may help prevent damage to DNA and decrease the risks of some cancers and illnesses such as atherosclerosis, diabetes, and Alzheimer's.

Studies also show that tart cherries may help decrease inflammation in joints and can even decrease muscle pain. Because of these findings, researchers are now trying to determine whether tart cherries can help individuals diagnosed with arthritis.

To gain the benefits of tart cherries, experts recommend consuming 8 to 12 ounces of tart cherry juice twice a day, morning and night. Also, you can buy the fruit, not just the juice.

Keep in mind that the cherry varieties commonly available in the produce section of grocery stores are sweet cherries, which are completely different both visually and in antioxidant composition. Tart cherries are usually dried or frozen. You can also find them in the pie-filling section of your grocery store; try to get tart cherries packed in water and then simply add them to your favorite smoothie, salad, or grain side dish.

Açaí Bowls

Prep time: 10 min • **Yield:** 2 servings

Ingredients	Directions
7 ounces frozen açaí pulp (look for a package like the one in Figure 14-1) **½ cup apple juice** **¼ cup unsweetened, refrigerated or boxed coconut milk** **2 medium bananas (1 frozen and 1 room temperature)** **6 medium strawberries, hulled and sliced** **¾ cup blueberries** **¼ cup gluten-free granola or Tart Cherry Muesli (see the preceding recipe)** **2 tablespoons honey**	**1** In a blender, combine the frozen açaí pulp, apple juice, coconut milk, and 1 frozen banana. Blend until smooth, adding more apple juice if needed. **2** Divide the frozen puree between two bowls. Top the blended mixture with slices of the remaining banana, strawberries, and blueberries. Sprinkle each bowl with granola. Prior to serving, drizzle the açaí bowls with honey.

Per serving: Calories 385 (From Fat 77); Fat 9g (Saturated 2g); Cholesterol 0mg; Sodium 17mg; Carbohydrate 77g (Dietary Fiber 9g); Protein 5g.

Vary It! Try almond, rice, cashew, or soy milk in place of coconut milk.

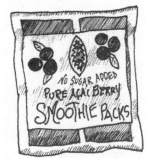

Figure 14-1:
Açaí pulp.

Illustration by Elizabeth Kurtzman

Lox and Rice Cakes

Prep time: 5 min • **Yield:** 4 servings

Ingredients	Directions
4 tablespoons capers, drained and rinsed	**1** In a small bowl, mix together the capers, red onion, lemon zest, and lemon juice with a fork.
2 tablespoons minced red onion	
1 medium lemon, zested and juiced (see Figure 14-2)	**2** Spread 1 tablespoon of labneh on each rice cake. Next, place 2 ounces of lox on each rice cake. Top with 1 tomato slice and 1 to 2 tablespoons of the caper mixture.
4 tablespoons labneh (kefir cheese)	
8 ounces lox (salmon), thinly sliced	
4 plain rice cakes	
1 Roma tomato, cut into 4 slices	

Per serving: Calories 119 (From Fat 30); Fat 3g (Saturated 1g); Cholesterol 13mg; Sodium 1,472mg; Carbohydrate 11g (Dietary Fiber 1g); Protein 13g.

Note: Capers are salty with a slight crunch to add texture and flavor to a recipe. They perfectly complement the smooth smokiness of the salmon. Caper berries or olives can be substituted in this recipe.

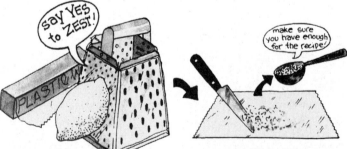

Figure 14-2: Zesting a lemon.

Cover the finest surface of the grater with plastic wrap.
Rub the citrus across the plastic-covered surface... (JUST THE COLORED PART! NOT THE BITTER WHITE PITH)!

say YES to ZEST!

make sure you have enough for the recipe!

When you think you've grated enough, lift off the plastic and scrape up the zest with a flat edge. Use a measuring spoon to see if you've grated enough.

Illustration by Elizabeth Kurtzman

Mushroom and Kale Frittata

Prep time: 2 min • **Cook time:** 30 min • **Yield:** 4 servings

Ingredients	Directions
2 tablespoons olive oil	*1* Preheat the oven to 400 degrees.
8 ounces mushrooms (button or cremini), sliced	*2* In a heavy, ovenproof 9-inch skillet (preferably cast iron), heat the olive oil over medium heat. Add the mushrooms and rosemary and sauté them for 10 minutes, or until the mushrooms are golden. Add the kale and sauté for an additional 3 minutes. Transfer the vegetables to a plate and wipe the skillet clean.
1 tablespoon minced fresh rosemary	
4 large kale leaves, stems removed, thinly sliced	
8 large eggs	*3* Whisk together the eggs, Greek yogurt, salt, and pepper in a large bowl. Add the cooked vegetables to the eggs.
2 tablespoons plain Greek yogurt	
¼ teaspoon salt	*4* Spray the pan with nonstick cooking spray (see the tip at the end of the recipe). Heat the skillet over medium-high heat. Pour the egg mixture into the skillet and cook for 2 minutes.
⅛ teaspoon black pepper	
2 ounces goat cheese, crumbled	*5* Top the eggs with the crumbled goat cheese and transfer the skillet to the oven. Bake for 12 to 15 minutes, or until the egg mixture is set in the center. (Jiggle the pan to see whether the egg mixture is set.)
	6 Allow the frittata to cool for 5 to 10 minutes prior to slicing it. Slice the frittata into four wedges and serve. Frittatas can be served hot or at room temperature.

Per serving: *Calories 271 (From Fat 180); Fat 20g (Saturated 7g); Cholesterol 390mg; Sodium 375mg; Carbohydrate 5g (Dietary Fiber 2g); Protein 19g.*

Vary It! Not a fan of mushrooms? Use eggplant, bell peppers, or grated carrots instead.

Tip: If you're concerned about using cooking spray, consider purchasing a pump mechanism where you pour in your oil of choice, pump with air, and spray.

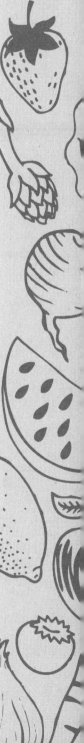

Huevos Rancheros

Prep time: 10 min • **Cook time:** 25 min • **Yield:** 4 servings

Ingredients	Directions
2 small tomatoes	*1* To prepare the salsa, put the tomatoes, onion, jalapeño, crushed garlic clove, ¼ cup cilantro, lime juice, and cumin in a food processor. Process the ingredients for 1 minute, or until they're completely pureed. Season the salsa with salt and pepper to taste.
1 small red onion	
1 medium jalapeño pepper, seeded (optional) and chopped	
2 cloves of garlic (1 crushed and 1 minced)	*2* Heat a medium skillet over low heat and add the 2 tablespoons olive oil. Fry the salsa in the oil until it thickens slightly, about 3 minutes. Put the salsa in a bowl and set it aside.
½ cup chopped cilantro, divided	
½ medium lime, juiced	*3* Add the beans to the same skillet along with the minced garlic, ½ cup warm water, and a pinch of salt. Cook over low heat, mixing slightly with a fork, until the beans are warmed through, about 5 minutes.
1 teaspoon ground cumin	
Kosher salt	
Freshly ground black pepper	
2 tablespoons olive oil, plus more for greasing the skillet	*4* Using a paper towel, wipe another medium skillet with olive oil. Heat the skillet over medium-high heat and warm the tortillas, one at a time, flipping the tortilla to warm each side. Keep the warm tortillas wrapped in a towel until it's time to assemble the dish.
15.5-ounce can refried black beans	
½ cup warm water	
1 to 2 teaspoons olive oil	*5* Wipe the skillet used for the tortillas with additional olive oil and heat the pan over medium heat. Fry the eggs according to your preferences.
Four 6-inch corn tortillas	
4 large eggs	*6* Put 1 warm tortilla on each plate. Divide the beans among the tortillas, and then top them each with a cooked egg and some salsa. Sprinkle with the remaining ¼ cup cilantro prior to serving.

Per serving: Calories 307 (From Fat 133); Fat 15g (Saturated 3g); Cholesterol 186mg; Sodium 351mg; Carbohydrate 30g (Dietary Fiber 8g); Protein 13g.

Breakfast Pho

Prep time: 25 min • **Cook time:** 20 min • **Yield:** 8 servings

Ingredients	Directions
1 pound thin rice noodles (vermicelli style, similar to angel hair)	*1* Soak the rice noodles in cold water for at least 20 minutes. Drain the noodles.
4 quarts organic, gluten-free beef or chicken broth	*2* Meanwhile, in a large stockpot, bring the broth to a full boil over medium heat. Add the liquid aminos, allspice, black pepper, cloves, cinnamon, and gingerroot. Lower the heat and allow the broth to simmer for 10 minutes.
¼ cup Bragg Liquid Aminos or coconut aminos	
1 teaspoon allspice	
1 teaspoon black pepper	*3* Divide the sliced green onions, cilantro, mint, basil, and bean sprouts among eight bowls.
¼ teaspoon ground cloves	
½ teaspoon ground cinnamon	
½ teaspoon chopped gingerroot	*4* Bring a large pot of water to a boil over medium-high heat. Then add the drained rice noodles. Give the noodles a quick stir and cook them until they're tender but firm, about 1 minute. Rice noodles can quickly become gummy, so don't let them overcook. Drain the noodles and divide them evenly among the eight bowls.
2 bunches green onions, sliced thin	
½ cup fresh cilantro, roughly chopped	
½ cup mint, roughly chopped	*5* Carefully ladle the simmering broth into the bowls and serve immediately. Garnish with lime wedges. Taste the broth and season with chili sauce or chilies as desired.
½ cup basil, roughly chopped	
1½ cups mung bean sprouts	
2 large limes, cut into wedges	
Sriracha (red chili sauce) or sliced fresh, hot chilies (optional)	

Per serving: Calories 260 (From Fat 20); Fat 2g (Saturated 0g); Cholesterol 10mg; Sodium 1,481mg; Carbohydrate 53g (Dietary Fiber 1g); Protein 7g.

Note: Although pho seems like an unusual breakfast, warm broth-based soups are popular in many cultures for breakfast. Something about starting your day with this flavorful soup is warming to the soul. Give it a try!

Tip: To store excess pho, place the broth in its own container, separate from the noodles, sprouts, herbs, and garnishes. To serve later, simply reheat the broth over medium-high heat. Put the other ingredients in your bowl and ladle the hot broth on top.

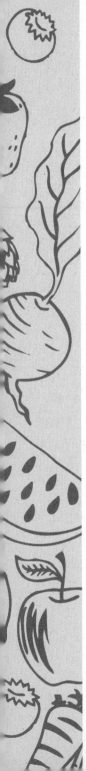

Note: Bragg Liquid Aminos is a certified non-GMO soybean product composed of 16 different amino acids; it tastes like soy sauce. Possibly harder to find but equally as notable are coconut aminos, which have 17 amino acids, are gluten-free and soy-free, and are organic.

Chapter 15

Enjoying Fuel-Filled Lunches

In This Chapter

▶ Getting a shot of protein

▶ Putting together lunches when you're on the go

*W*hipping into a fast food restaurant may be a simple solution for lunch, but if fast food is part of your regular "nutrition plan," you're slowly destroying your health with overprocessed and nutrient-deficient food. It's time to break the habit of drive-throughs and focus on convenient foods that heal.

Wait — did we say "convenient" and "foods that heal" in the same sentence? Yes! Foods in their simplest forms, without refinement and processing, can be the most healing, especially for folks with adrenal fatigue. Nothing is less refined than an apple fresh off the tree or a carrot plucked from the soil. You don't even need to plant a garden to attain these benefits. Stocking your pantry and refrigerator with the right foods can show you that lunch really is convenient.

Numerous cultures make lunch their largest meal of the day. Don't fret if this doesn't fit into your schedule; instead, find a pattern that works for you and your body. Whatever you do, remember to eat — lunch is critical, not to be missed. This chapter guides you on the best ways to get a protein boost and to pack on-the-go lunches. It features some tasty recipes that are perfect for lunch. *Note:* Recipes listed with a tomato icon are vegetarian.

Powering Up with Protein

Protein creates *satiety* (feeling satisfied after consuming food), builds lean muscle, and provides essential nutrients to help a fatigued body repair itself. Fish, meats, poultry, eggs, and dairy are some of the best protein-rich foods. Some plant-based foods, such as beans, whole grains, nuts, and seeds, are also excellent protein sources. Whatever you choose, try to get at least 30 grams of protein at each meal. Here's what 30 grams looks like:

- 5 ounces salmon
- 4 ounces (1 small) chicken breast
- 3 ounces lean sirloin steak
- 5 boiled eggs
- 2 cups lentils
- 5 ounces almonds
- 2 cups broccoli + 1.5 cups kefir
- 1 to 2 scoops whey protein powder

Boiling eggs

One essential kitchen skill everyone should have is hard-boiling an egg. Eggs are a perfect source of protein for humans and a great source of vitamin D. In addition, you can add boiled eggs to any salad. You can also eat them on the go, because they're naturally protected by their shell (thus eliminating storage needs). In essence, a boiled egg is a great asset to your refrigerator and your diet.

To hard-boil eggs, place the raw eggs in a saucepan and cover them with cold tap water. Be sure the eggs aren't crammed in and that none are on top of each other. Next, bring the water to a boil over medium-high heat. When the water reaches a full boil, remove the pot from the heat source and cover the pot for 13 minutes. Immediately drain the eggs and run cold water over them for 3 minutes to halt the cooking process. You can store boiled eggs in the refrigerator for up to one week.

Remember: The yolk boasts key nutrients such as vitamin D and choline, so be sure to enjoy the whole egg, not just the white!

Keeping Lunch Simple

If you're like a lot of folks, your work schedule may make finding time for lunch one of the most stressful parts of your day. But it's critical to step away from your work and give your mind a break as you nourish yourself and reboot your energy for the afternoon. (See Chapter 13 for some tips on getting the most out of your lunch break.)

For the days that seem to get away from you, be sure to keep things simple. Here are some time-saving meals to pick up, keep on hand, or toss together:

- ✔ Premade salads (look for dark, bold greens or cabbages)
- ✔ Sushi rolls (stay simple and ditch the sauces)
- ✔ Leftovers (how about from the recipes in this chapter and in Chapter 16?)
- ✔ Organic soups
- ✔ Rice cakes with almond butter
- ✔ Tuna salad served in an avocado
- ✔ Cottage cheese, sunflower seeds, and chopped vegetables

A power lunch tray (see Figure 15-1) is a great option for a simple meal. When you're creating your personal power lunch box, be sure to pick at least three different nutrient-packed items, and alternate choices from one day to the next. Choose three or more of the following to create a combo:

- ✔ **Fast fats:** Avocado, mixed nuts and seeds, olives
- ✔ **Cruciferous crunch:** Broccoli, cauliflower, shredded cabbage
- ✔ **Dips:** Greek yogurt, hummus, bean dip, nut butter, olive tapenade
- ✔ **Digestive fruits (with digestive enzymes):** Papaya, mango, pineapple
- ✔ **Fruity fiber:** Raspberries, blackberries, strawberries, blueberries
- ✔ **Citrus craze:** Clementines (mandarin oranges), kumquats, blood oranges
- ✔ **Powerful protein:** Sirloin steak, chicken breast, turkey meatballs

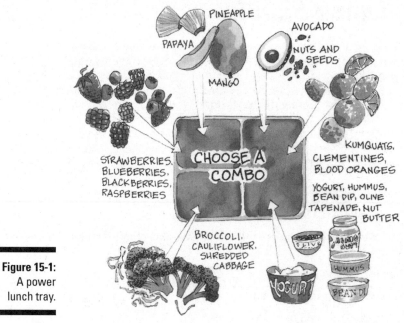

Figure 15-1:
A power
lunch tray.

Choose a variety of nutrient-dense foods and vary them from day to day. Create balance in your meal with lean proteins and satiating fats, and when you're craving something sweet, tune in to the sweetness of an apple or fresh strawberries instead of grabbing a candy bar. Consider complementing your meal with a gluten-free grain salad, a fruit salad, satisfying greens, or a bean burger. At each meal, include something basic and unrefined, such as raw fruits and vegetables. Break the addiction to processed foods by focusing on whole foods for satisfaction and health.

Broiled Avocados

Prep time: 5 min • **Cook time:** 7 min • **Yield:** 4 servings

Ingredients	Directions
2 medium avocados, sliced in half and pitted (see Figure 15-2)	*1* Set the top oven rack about 5 inches away from the heating element. Preheat the broiler.
1 medium lime **1 tablespoon chia seeds** **4 tablespoons goat cheese, crumbled**	*2* Place the avocado halves on a baking sheet, cut side up. Cut the lime in half and squeeze lime juice over the avocados. Sprinkle the avocados with chia seeds and goat cheese.
¼ cup chopped cilantro	*3* Broil the avocados for 5 to 7 minutes, or until the cheese melts and is slightly golden. Top the broiled avocados with fresh cilantro prior to serving.

Per serving: Calories 172 (From Fat 136); Fat 15g (Saturated 4g); Cholesterol 9mg; Sodium 35mg; Carbohydrate 10g (Dietary Fiber 9g); Protein 4g.

Note: Chia seeds are little black seeds from the plant *Salvia hispanica.* They're gaining popularity due to their omega-3, fiber, and protein content. Unlike flaxseeds, chia seeds don't require milling for you to reap the health benefits. They're mild in flavor and add a slight crunch to any dish.

How to Pit and Peel an Avocado

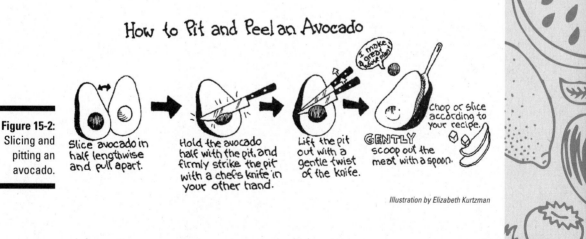

Figure 15-2: Slicing and pitting an avocado.

Slice avocado in half lengthwise and pull apart.

Hold the avocado half with the pit, and firmly strike the pit with a chef's knife in your other hand.

Lift the pit out with a gentle twist of the knife.

GENTLY scoop out the meat with a spoon.

Chop or slice according to your recipe.

Illustration by Elizabeth Kurtzman

Creamy Broccoli Salad

Prep time: 15 min • 1 hr • **Yield:** 8 servings

Ingredients	Directions
6 cups chopped broccoli crowns	**1** In a large mixing bowl, stir together the chopped broccoli and apple cider vinegar. Add the grated carrots, cherries, sunflower seeds, and mandarin oranges. Mix well.
1 tablespoon apple cider vinegar	
¾ cup grated carrots	
½ cup dried tart cherries	**2** Fold the Greek yogurt into the mixture until the salad is thoroughly combined. Allow the salad to chill in the refrigerator for at least 1 hour before serving.
½ cup shelled, roasted sunflower seeds	
½ cup canned mandarin oranges	
1½ cups plain Greek yogurt	

Per serving: Calories 130 (From Fat 44); Fat 5g (Saturated 1g); Cholesterol 3mg; Sodium 39mg; Carbohydrate 15g (Dietary Fiber 3g); Protein 8g.

Tip: The flavors really come together if you refrigerate the salad overnight.

Kinky Kale Salad

Prep time: 8 min • **Yield:** 4 servings

Ingredients	Directions
12 ounces kale, stems removed and leaves cut into thin slices (about 4 cups); see Figure 15-3	*1* Place the kale in a large mixing bowl and drizzle it with apple cider vinegar. Use your hands to massage the kale, watching as the color brightens! Remove the brightened greens and place them in a large serving bowl.
¼ cup apple cider vinegar	
1 tablespoon miso paste (preferably mild yellow miso)	*2* Make a vinaigrette by whisking together the miso paste, lemon juice, liquid aminos, olive oil, and sesame oil (if desired). Toss the kale with the vinaigrette and serve the salad with almonds.
1 medium lemon, juiced	
2 teaspoons Bragg Liquid Aminos or coconut aminos	
2 teaspoons extra virgin olive oil	
1 teaspoon sesame oil (optional)	
½ cup whole, chopped, or sliced almonds	

Per serving: Calories 170 (From Fat 108); Fat 12g (Saturated 1g); Cholesterol 0mg; Sodium 297mg; Carbohydrate 12g (Dietary Fiber 4g); Protein 7g.

Note: You can find Bragg Liquid Aminos at most grocery stores or health food stores. This product, which boasts 16 amino acids, is a gluten-free substitute for soy sauce. If you're sensitive to soy, consider trying coconut aminos.

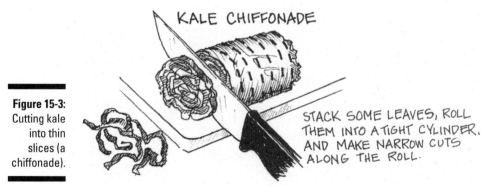

KALE CHIFFONADE

STACK SOME LEAVES, ROLL THEM INTO A TIGHT CYLINDER, AND MAKE NARROW CUTS ALONG THE ROLL.

Figure 15-3: Cutting kale into thin slices (a chiffonade).

Illustration by Elizabeth Kurtzman

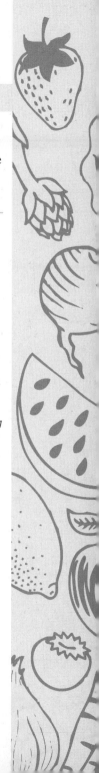

Tropical Fruit Salad

Prep time: 15 min • **Yield:** 8 servings

Ingredients	Directions
1 medium mango, peeled, pitted, and cubed	**1** Toss the mango, pineapple, papaya, and kiwi fruit in a large serving bowl. Top the fruit with coconut flakes and macadamia nuts.
1 pineapple, cubed (approximately 4 cups)	
1 cup cubed papaya	**2** Stir together the lime juice and honey in a small microwave-safe bowl and cook on full power for 10 seconds (or warm the mixture on the stovetop in a small saucepan). Stir the honey-lime sauce and then drizzle it over the fruit. Toss the salad before serving.
2 medium kiwis, peeled and cubed	
¼ cup unsweetened coconut flakes	
¼ cup macadamia nuts, chopped	
1 medium lime, juiced	
2 tablespoons honey	

Per serving: Calories 168 (From Fat 49); Fat 6g (Saturated 2g); Cholesterol 0mg; Sodium 4mg; Carbohydrate 32g (Dietary Fiber 4g); Protein 2g.

Note: You can use cored, fresh pineapple from the refrigerator section of your grocery store instead of cutting up a whole pineapple.

Black Bean Burgers

Prep time: 20 min • **Cook time:** 8 min • **Yield:** 4 servings

Ingredients	Directions
15-ounce can black beans, drained and rinsed **½ cup minced red onion** **½ cup gluten-free oats** **¼ cup chopped cilantro** **2 teaspoons minced jalapeño** **¼ teaspoon salt** **1 medium egg** **1 tablespoon yellow cornmeal** **¼ cup olive oil** **1 cup salsa**	**1** In a food processor, combine the black beans, red onion, oats, cilantro, jalapeño, salt, and egg. Pulse the mixture until the ingredients are just combined, about 1 minute total. **2** Take the black bean mixture out of food processor and form four patties about ½ inch thick. Dredge each side of the black bean patties in the cornmeal and set them aside. **3** In a large, heavy skillet (preferably cast iron), heat the olive oil over medium-high heat. Cook each patty for 4 minutes on each side. Serve with salsa.

Per serving: Calories 285 (From Fat 139); Fat 16g (Saturated 2g); Cholesterol 0mg; Sodium 762mg; Carbohydrate 28g (Dietary Fiber 9g); Protein 10g.

Tip: A typical can of black beans (15 ounces) has 400 milligrams of added sodium. That's 114 milligrams per serving! Draining and then rinsing your beans can cut sodium by 41 percent, so don't skip that step. Or instead of using canned beans, consider cooking dried black beans the night before.

Vary It! Any bean variety can work here, so get creative with pinto beans, white beans, or lentils.

Tip: These bean burgers are great to freeze. You can wrap them in foil and freeze them for up to a month. No need to defrost; just bake the frozen patties at 350 degrees for 20 minutes or pan-fry them for 8 minutes on each side.

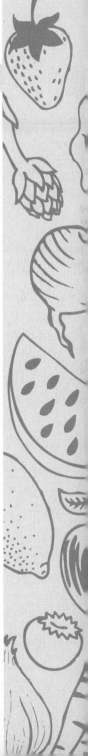

Curried Lentil Salad

Prep time: 8 min • **Cook time:** 30 min • **Yield:** 4 servings

Ingredients	Directions
2 cups water	*1* In a 2-quart saucepan, bring the water and lentils to a boil over high heat. Reduce the heat to low and simmer for 30 minutes, or until the lentils are tender. Drain.
1 cup dry brown lentils	
1 cup frozen peas, defrosted	
3 Roma tomatoes, chopped	*2* In a medium serving bowl, mix together the lentils, peas, tomatoes, and carrot.
1 medium carrot, grated	
1 medium lemon, juiced	*3* In a small bowl, whisk together the lemon juice, curry powder, and olive oil. Stir the lemon dressing into the salad.
1 teaspoon curry powder	
2 tablespoons olive oil	
½ cup chopped fresh cilantro	*4* Top the salad with chopped cilantro and serve. Season with salt, as desired. This salad is excellent chilled or at room temperature.
Salt	

Per serving: Calories 274 (From Fat 67); Fat 8g (Saturated 1g); Cholesterol 0mg; Sodium 341mg; Carbohydrate 39g (Dietary Fiber 15g); Protein 15g.

Tip: If you have fresh turmeric or ginger on hand, grate it finely and stir it in with the curry powder! Start with a small amount and work up to your taste preference.

Millet and Miso Stuffed Tomato Bites

Prep time: 10 min • **Cook time:** 20 min • **Yield:** 10 servings

Ingredients	Directions
2 cups chicken or vegetable stock	*1* In a 2-quart saucepan, combine the stock and millet. Heat the mixture to a boil over medium-high heat. Reduce the heat to low, cover the pan, and cook the millet until all the water is absorbed, about 15 minutes.
1 cup millet	
4 green onions, chopped	
2 cups chopped parsley	*2* In a large mixing bowl, combine the cooked millet, green onions, parsley, pine nuts, and feta.
½ cup pine nuts	
¼ cup crumbled feta cheese (from goat's milk or sheep's milk)	*3* In a small mixing bowl, whisk together the lemon zest, lemon juice, miso, chia seeds, and olive oil. Drizzle the lemon dressing over the millet and mix thoroughly.
2 medium lemons, zested and juiced	
1 tablespoon miso paste	
3 tablespoons chia seeds	*4* Cut each tomato in half lengthwise and hollow out the tomato halves. Spoon the millet into the tomato halves and serve.
½ cup olive oil	
15 medium Roma tomatoes	

Per serving: Calories 274 (From Fat 165); Fat 19g (Saturated 3g); Cholesterol 0mg; Sodium 306mg; Carbohydrate 23g (Dietary Fiber 5g); Protein 6g.

Note: Millet — not just for the birds! This gluten-free seed is a great grain alternative with a mildly sweet taste and nutty texture.

Note: This recipe yields ten servings, but leftovers hold up well all week. When you make these tomato bites, make a lot and make them last!

Beet and Orange Quinoa Salad

Prep time: 5 min • **Cook time:** 20 min • **Chill time:** 30 min • **Yield:** 8 servings

Ingredients	Directions
2 cups water	**1** In a 2-quart saucepan, bring 2 cups water to a boil over high heat. Add the quinoa, reduce the heat to low, cover the pan, and allow the quinoa to simmer for 15 minutes, or until it's fluffy.
1 cup quinoa, rinsed	
3 medium oranges, peeled and cubed	
2 cups shredded raw beets (include the peeling but discard the greens and root stem)	**2** In a mixing bowl, stir together the oranges, beets, green onions, pine nuts, and navy beans. Stir in the cooked quinoa.
1 cup chopped green onions	
¼ cup pine nuts	**3** In a separate bowl, make a vinaigrette by whisking together the red wine vinegar, Dijon mustard, garlic, and salt to taste. Pour the vinaigrette over the quinoa/ vegetable mixture and stir. Chill the salad for at least 30 minutes before serving.
15-ounce can navy beans, drained and rinsed	
2 tablespoons red wine vinegar	
1 teaspoon Dijon mustard	
2 cloves garlic, minced	
Salt	

Per serving: Calories 204 (From Fat 44); Fat 5g (Saturated 0g); Cholesterol 0mg; Sodium 216mg; Carbohydrate 35g (Dietary Fiber 11g); Protein 8g.

Note: Quinoa is an ancient gluten-free seed that has gained popularity due to its high-quality protein and fiber content.

Tip: If you can't shred the beets in a food processor, grate them manually using a cheese grater (see Figure 15-4). Be sure to wear an apron or clothing that isn't valuable, because beet stains can be difficult to remove.

Vary It! You can use fresh parsley, sunflower seeds, or red onion in place of green onions or pine nuts. You can also substitute canned mandarin oranges (packed in water, not syrup) for fresh oranges.

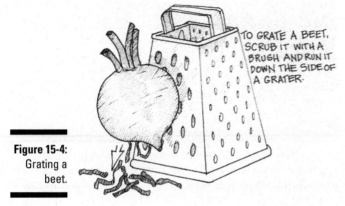

Figure 15-4:
Grating a
beet.

Illustration by Elizabeth Kurtzman

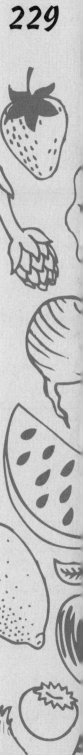

Southwestern Steak and Sweet Potato Salad

Prep time: 35 min • **Cook time:** 20 min • **Yield:** 4 servings

Ingredients	Directions
1 large sweet potato (about 8 to 12 ounces)	**1** Place the sweet potato in a medium saucepan and add enough cold water to cover the sweet potato. Bring the water to a boil over high heat. Reduce the heat to low, cover the pot, and simmer for 20 minutes, or until the sweet potato is fork-tender. Drain off the water and run the sweet potato under cold water to halt the cooking process. Set the sweet potato aside to cool.
2 medium limes, zested and juiced	
½ cup olive oil	
¼ cup chopped cilantro	
1 clove garlic, minced	**2** While the sweet potato cooks, make a vinaigrette by mixing together the lime zest, lime juice, olive oil, cilantro, garlic, and red onion. Season the vinaigrette with salt to taste and set it aside.
¼ cup minced red onion	
Salt	
12 to 16 ounces sirloin steak	**3** Slice the steak into ½-inch strips. Heat a large skillet over medium-high heat, add the steak, and cook it for 3 minutes on each side. Remove the steak from the skillet and lightly season it with salt and pepper.
Black pepper	
8 cups green leaf or red leaf lettuce, washed and torn	
2 tablespoons pumpkin seeds, with or without shells	**4** Place the lettuce greens on a large platter. Cut the cooked sweet potato into cubes and sprinkle it over lettuce greens. Lay the steak strips over the lettuce and drizzle the vinaigrette over the top.
	5 Finish the salad with a sprinkle of pumpkin seeds prior to serving.

Per serving: Calories 468 (From Fat 317); Fat 36g (Saturated 7g); Cholesterol 56mg; Sodium 242mg; Carbohydrate 16g (Dietary Fiber 4g); Protein 22g.

Vary It! Chicken breast or thighs taste great in place of the sirloin steak.

Chapter 16

Tuning In to Dinnertime

Dinner can be a wonderful part of your day, as unwinding around a flavorful and nourishing meal helps you destress. Don't worry — preparing a good dinner can be easy and fun. The recipes in this chapter are packed with antioxidants and healing nutrients to help your body repair itself and boost your energy; they also satisfy your hunger as you tune in to your body and what you're eating. *Note:* The recipe listed with a tomato icon is vegetarian.

Getting Powerful Nutrients at Dinner

A simple guideline for an evening meal is to fill half of your plate with brightly colored vegetables and match them with 3 to 5 ounces of lean protein and ½ to 1 cup of gluten-free grains. Here are some example combinations:

✔ 2 cups steamed broccoli, 4 ounces sirloin steak, and ½ cup rice

✔ Half of a cabbage head, braised, with 5 ounces grilled salmon and ½ cup quinoa

✔ 2 cups salad with 5 ounces grilled chicken breast and ¾ cup black beans

For good health — especially if you have adrenal fatigue — pack your dinners with nutrient-dense vegetables and lean proteins to provide the arsenal your body needs to heal and mend overnight.

Fixing dinner without the stress

Making dinner doesn't need to add to the stress of your day-to-day life. With a little preparation and planning, you can be in and out of the kitchen in 30 minutes. Here are some ideas for making dinner without the stress:

✔ Stock your refrigerator and pantry with healthy staples (like the ones found in this book).

✔ Buy chopped vegetables to shorten prep work.

✔ Make double batches to carry over food for the next night.

✔ After cooking, consider freezing half of the food to enjoy another day.

Eating Mindfully at Dinner

Perhaps you've heard of *mindful* or *intuitive eating.* Authors Brian Wansink and Evelyn Tribole are pioneering the way toward teaching people how to eat "normally." Forcing yourself to eat when you're not really hungry isn't normal. Neither is skipping a meal when you'd rather eat.

Recognizing unhealthy relationships with food

To see what normal eating is, watch a young child eat. When the child is no longer hungry, he or she turns away or pushes the food away. Now, what do parents typically do? They plead with their child, "One more bite, one more bite." This practice begins counteracting the child's instinct to stop eating when he or she is satisfied.

Many people claim to put on their "fat pants" (insert cringe) before they go out for a big meal. Or they plan to "eat their weight in gold" for a special occasion. This isn't good, either. Why eat beyond hunger? Does it really feel good? Overeating doesn't create long-lasting pleasure or satisfaction. In fact, it makes you feel slow, sluggish, and even sick. Over time, it causes you to gain weight, and even a couple of added pounds can further fatigue the adrenals and increase joint pain.

Consider emotional reactions to overindulgence, too: guilt, excuses, and self-degrading comments. These reactions do nothing but negate a healthy relationship with food. If you have adrenal fatigue, you don't want negative emotions that might contribute to depression.

Here are just a few ways you may curtail your natural ability to say, "Hey, I'm full and don't need to eat any more."

- ✔ Skipping meals and then feasting after the famine
- ✔ Eating beyond the point of feeling comfortable
- ✔ Saving up for one big meal per day
- ✔ Using big plates and feeling as though you must eat everything on it

Being aware of your food and your body

The following practices can get you started on a path to mindful eating, both at dinner and throughout the day:

- ✔ Listen to your body and eat when you're hungry.

- ✔ Before you start eating, ask yourself, "Am I hungry?" If not, drop the fork and go do something else. (Or if you want to indulge in something special, savor just a few bites — see Chapter 17 for details on the three-bite rule.)

- ✔ If you're full or no longer hungry, give yourself permission to stop eating.

Sitting down to a good meal

What does the dinner table mean to you? Is it a place to pay bills? Fold laundry? Stack papers? Or is it a place where people gather only during holidays or special occasions? For day-to-day dinners, do you insist on sitting at the table anymore? Research shows that distractions lead to overeating and indigestion, which aren't good for anyone, especially folks with adrenal fatigue.

Bring back the tradition of sitting while you eat! The point of the dinner table is to bring family and friends together and to give you a place to eat and unwind as you decrease the clutter on your mind. The simple act of sitting down at a meal helps you tune in to what you're enjoying (why rush a good meal?), aids in digestion by slowing you down, and allows you to tune out stressful aspects of your day. If you have adrenal fatigue, these benefits are doubly important. You want to reduce stress and increase your appreciation for the foods you're eating (some of which may be new to you).

✔ Recognize which foods truly make you feel good and which ones give you temporary joy but leave you feeling guilty later.

✔ Ditch the 14-inch dinner plates. Try using 9-inch dinner plates or salad plates. The portions will look bigger.

✔ Sit down at a dinner table to eat, free of distractions. You can't focus on the food if you're watching TV or texting.

✔ When you're eating, really taste your food. Focus on texture, aroma, and flavor as you savor each bite.

You really have to retrain yourself to become a more mindful eater. Read *Intuitive Eating* (published by St. Martin's Griffin) by Evelyn Tribole, MS, RD, and Elyse Resch, MS, RD, FADA, CEDRD, for a new approach to eating and breaking the destructive dieting cycle.

Don't toss out the zest!

If you really want a powerful citrus flavor, look no further than the peel. Not only is citrus peel flavorful, but it's packed with polymethoxylated flavones (PMFs), which may help lower cholesterol and help prevent diabetes. In addition, the peel has high levels of antioxidants, including vitamin C. Adding zest to your food is a simple means to increase flavor and antioxidants to support the adrenals.

Invest in a microplane or a conventional zester and watch your food transform. Be sure not to zest down to the white rind (the pith). Instead, gently remove the outer portion of the peel, where all the flavor hides. Adding zest to beverages also adds flavor without giving you reason to worry about gut issues.

Whether in finishing sauces, brightening salads, or transforming desserts, people use citrus zest daily throughout the world. If you don't know where to begin, here are some simple uses for citrus zest:

✔ Zest is a perfect addition to any salad dressing. You can also zest a lemon, lime, orange, or grapefruit over the top of a tossed salad.

✔ Add the zest to your water to infuse it with flavor.

✔ If you're making scones or muffins, add a bit of citrus zest to wow your taste buds.

✔ Finish preparing a grain salad with some zest for a pop of color and flavor.

If you find yourself with an abundant supply of citrus, place the zest in ice cube trays. Cover the zest with water or juice and freeze. Then you're ready to add the cubes to your favorite juice, stock, water, or cocktail.

Spaghetti Squash with Pesto Chicken

Prep time: 15 min • **Cook time:** 35 min • **Yield:** 4 servings

Ingredients	Directions
1 medium spaghetti squash (about 2.5 pounds), halved, seeds removed	*1* Preheat the oven to 425 degrees.
1 cup water	*2* Place the spaghetti squash halves on a rimmed baking sheet, cut side down. Add the water to the pan (this prevents sticking and helps steam the spaghetti squash). Bake for 20 to 25 minutes, or until the spaghetti squash is easy to pierce with a fork. To create spaghetti-like threads, handle the spaghetti squash with a heat-resistant glove or towel and scrape the flesh out with a fork (see Figure 16-1).
1 tablespoon plus ½ cup olive oil	
1 pound boneless, skinless chicken breasts, cut into ¼-inch slices	
½ cup pine nuts	*3* In a heavy skillet, heat 1 tablespoon olive oil over medium-high heat and sauté the chicken for 5 to 7 minutes, or until it's cooked completely. Remove the skillet from the heat.
2 cups basil leaves	
2 garlic cloves	
1 medium lemon, juiced	*4* In a food processor, add the pine nuts, basil, garlic, and lemon juice. Pulse the mixture for a total of 1 minute. Then slowly drizzle the remaining ½ cup olive oil into the mixture while blending. Stop adding oil when the mixture looks creamy. Season the pesto with salt according to taste.
Salt	
	5 In a serving bowl, toss together the spaghetti squash threads, sautéed chicken, and pesto sauce before serving.

Per serving: Calories 578 (From Fat 403); Fat 45g (Saturated 6g); Cholesterol 63mg; Sodium 245mg; Carbohydrate 20g (Dietary Fiber 4g); Protein 28g.

Vary It! Top this dish with ½ cup sun-dried tomatoes for a pop of color and a nutritional boost.

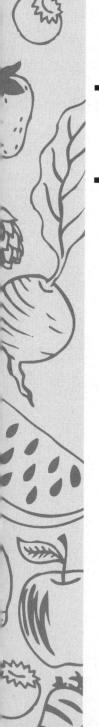

CUTTING AND STRINGING SPAGHETTI SQUASH

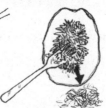

Figure 16-1:
Cutting and
stringing a
spaghetti
squash.

1. USE A CHEF'S KNIFE TO CUT THE SQUASH IN HALF LENGTH-WISE. SCOOP OUT THE SEEDS WITH A SPOON.

2. COOK THE SQUASH, AND THEN USE A FORK TO SCRAPE OUT THE FLESH AND CREATE STRINGS. BE CAREFUL NOT TO BREAK THROUGH THE END.

Illustration by Elizabeth Kurtzman

Chicken, Kale, and Garbanzo Curry

Prep time: 5 min • **Cook time:** 18 min • **Yield:** 4 servings

Ingredients	Directions
4 boneless chicken thighs (about 1 pound total), skin removed	*1* Coat a nonstick skillet with cooking spray. Over medium-high heat, cook the chicken thighs on both sides (about 4 to 5 minutes each side).
14.5-ounce can garbanzo beans, drained and rinsed	*2* Remove the cooked chicken from the skillet. When the chicken is cool, cut it into bite-sized pieces.
2 tablespoons curry powder	
2 cloves garlic, minced	*3* Add the garbanzo beans, curry powder, and garlic to the skillet and cook them for 3 minutes over medium heat, stirring gently every 20 to 30 seconds.
4 large kale leaves, stems removed, thinly sliced (see Chapter 15 for pointers on slicing kale)	
¼ cup apple cider vinegar	*4* Add the kale and cooked chicken to the skillet and cook over medium heat for 4 to 5 minutes, until the kale is softened and bright green.
1 cup canned coconut milk	
1 pinch red pepper flakes	*5* Add the apple cider vinegar and the canned coconut milk to the mixture in the skillet. Stir well and then simmer for 2 minutes.
Salt	
	6 Season with red pepper flakes and salt to taste.

Per serving: Calories 372 (From Fat 188); Fat 21g (Saturated 13g); Cholesterol 106mg; Sodium 380mg; Carbohydrate 22g (Dietary Fiber 1g); Protein 26g.

Note: Concerned with using cooking sprays? Consider purchasing a pump mechanism where you pour in your oil of choice, pump with air, and spray.

Salmon with Olive Tapenade over Wilted Spinach

Prep time: 8 min • **Cook time:** 30 min • **Yield:** 6 servings

Ingredients	Directions
2 pounds salmon (preferably wild Alaskan with skin on)	*1* Preheat the oven to 400 degrees.
¼ teaspoon salt	*2* Spray a 9-x-13-inch pan with nonstick cooking spray. Place the fish in the pan and season the fish with salt and pepper. Bake for 25 to 30 minutes, or until the fish flakes easily with a fork.
¼ teaspoon black pepper	
1 cup Kalamata olives, pitted	
½ cup fresh parsley	
2 tablespoons capers, drained	*3* While the fish is cooking, add the olives, parsley, capers, and 2 tablespoons of olive oil to the bowl of your food processor. Pulse the olive mixture until it's smooth.
4 tablespoons olive oil, divided	
6 cloves garlic, thinly sliced	*4* Before the fish finishes cooking, heat the remaining 2 tablespoons of olive oil in a large skillet over medium heat. Add the garlic and spinach. Cook and toss the garlic and spinach until the spinach is slightly wilted, about 2 to 3 minutes.
10 ounces fresh baby spinach	
4 tablespoons labneh (kefir cheese)	
	5 To assemble and serve this dish, place the wilted spinach on six plates, top it with baked fish, and finish with the olive mixture and a dollop of Labneh over each portion.

Per serving: Calories 347 (From Fat 180); Fat 20g (Saturated 3g); Cholesterol 71mg; Sodium 686mg; Carbohydrate 9g (Dietary Fiber 3g); Protein 33g.

Note: You can use a strained Greek yogurt in place of labneh; however, Greek yogurt has fewer bacteria strains. Using labneh, also known as *kefir cheese,* is a great way to boost your diet with a variety of probiotics (see Chapter 11). Most kefirs are prepared with at least 7 different strains of bacteria!

Mushroom and Kale Stroganoff

Prep time: 5 min • **Cook time:** 25 min • **Yield:** 2 servings

Ingredients	Directions
1 cup water	**1** In a 2-quart saucepan, bring the water to a boil over high heat. Add the rice. When the water returns to a boil, cover and simmer the rice for 25 minutes, or until the water is absorbed.
½ cup basmati rice, rinsed	
1 tablespoon olive oil	
½ medium white onion, thinly sliced	**2** Meanwhile, in a large skillet, heat the olive oil over medium-high heat. Add the onions and sauté them for 4 minutes. Add the mushrooms and garlic and sauté them for 15 minutes.
1 pound button or cremini mushrooms, rinsed and quartered	
3 cloves garlic, minced	**3** Add the miso, tahini, and liquid aminos to the skillet and stir gently. Add the vegetable broth and bring the mixture to a boil over medium heat.
2 teaspoons yellow miso	
1 tablespoon tahini	
2 teaspoons Bragg Liquid Aminos or coconut aminos	**4** Stir in the kale, cover the skillet, and remove it from the heat.
1 cup gluten-free vegetable broth	**5** Place the cooked rice in a serving bowl, spoon mushroom stroganoff on top, and sprinkle with thyme.
5 large kale leaves, stems removed, thinly sliced (see Chapter 15 for pointers)	
1 tablespoon minced fresh thyme	

Per serving: Calories 394 (From Fat 104); Fat 12g (Saturated 2g); Cholesterol 0mg; Sodium 754mg; Carbohydrate 65g (Dietary Fiber 6g); Protein 15g.

Note: Bragg Liquid Aminos is a gluten-free combination of essential amino acids made into a liquid that tastes similar to soy sauce. You can use coconut aminos instead if you're sensitive to soy-based products. Braggs Liquid Aminos can be found at most grocery stores or health food markets.

Note: Tahini is a sesame paste often found in Mediterranean markets or the nut butter aisle of a grocery store.

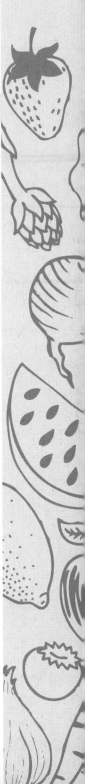

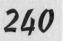

Chicken Tortilla Soup

Prep time: 20 min • **Cook time:** 30 min • **Yield:** 4 servings

Ingredients	Directions
2 quarts low-sodium chicken broth	**1** In a 4-quart saucepan over medium heat, cook the chicken broth, chicken breasts, diced tomatoes (with juice), diced tomatoes with green chilies (with juice), cumin, and coriander for 30 minutes.
2 large chicken breasts (about 1.5 pounds)	
14.5-ounce can diced tomatoes	**2** Remove the chicken from the saucepan. When the chicken is cool, dice it or shred it with two forks. Then return the chicken to the saucepan.
10-ounce can diced tomatoes with green chilies	
2 teaspoons cumin	**3** In a medium bowl, gently stir together the avocados (do not mash), onion, jalapeño, cilantro, and lime juice. Season the avocado mixture with salt to taste.
½ teaspoon coriander	
2 medium avocados, diced	
¼ medium red onion, diced	**4** In each of four serving bowls, place six corn tortilla chips. Top the chips with the avocado mixture and then ladle soup over the top and serve.
1 small jalapeño, minced	
1 cup chopped cilantro	
2 medium limes, juiced	
Salt	
24 corn tortilla chips	

Per serving: Calories 453 (From Fat 169); Fat 19g (Saturated 3g); Cholesterol 94mg; Sodium 932mg; Carbohydrate 28g (Dietary Fiber 6g); Protein 44g.

Note: If you're sensitive to the heat of the jalapeños, consider wearing gloves while you work with them. Also, feel free to adjust amount of jalapeño according to your heat preference.

Turkey Vegetable Lasagna

Prep time: 35 min • **Cook time:** 1 hr, 10 min • **Yield:** 8 servings

Ingredients	Directions
1 pound ground turkey breast	**1** Preheat the oven to 375 degrees.
1 pound white button mushrooms, sliced	**2** In a 10-inch sauté pan, brown the ground turkey and mushrooms until they're fully cooked, about 10 minutes.
1 clove garlic, sliced (or ½ teaspoon garlic powder)	
3 tablespoons chopped parsley, divided	**3** In a stockpot, combine the garlic, 1 tablespoon parsley, basil, tomatoes, tomato paste, and 1½ teaspoons salt. Simmer the tomato mixture over medium-low heat for 30 minutes. Add the ground turkey and mushrooms to the sauce.
1 tablespoon chopped basil	
28-ounce can diced tomatoes	
Two 6-ounce cans tomato paste	
3½ teaspoons salt, divided	**4** While the sauce is cooking, heat a grill pan over medium-high heat. Cook the zucchini for 2 to 3 minutes on each side.
6 large zucchinis, cut lengthwise into ⅛-inch slices	
3 cups cream-style cottage cheese or ricotta cheese	**5** In a mixing bowl, combine the cottage cheese, the eggs, the remaining 2 tablespoons parsley, the Parmesan cheese, the remaining 2 teaspoons salt, and the pepper.
2 eggs, beaten	
½ cup grated Parmesan cheese	**6** Spread a layer of the sauce across the bottom of a 9-x-13-inch baking pan, and then layer half of the grilled zucchini, half of the cottage cheese mixture, and half of the tomato sauce. Repeat the layers using the other half of the ingredients.
½ teaspoon black pepper	
	7 Bake for 30 minutes. Remove the lasagna from the oven and allow it to rest for 15 minutes before serving.

Per serving: *Calories 290 (From Fat 64); Fat 7g (Saturated 0g); Cholesterol 99mg; Sodium 1,689mg; Carbohydrate 25g (Dietary Fiber 5g); Protein 35g.*

Tip: Cooking for a smaller group? Consider baking this lasagna in three bread pans and freezing two for later.

Spicy Chicken and Coconut Soup

Prep time: 20 min • **Cook time:** 35 min • **Yield:** 4 servings

Ingredients	*Directions*
1 tablespoon olive oil	*1* In a 4-quart saucepan, heat the olive oil over medium-high heat. Add the chicken pieces and brown for 3 minutes.
1 pound boneless, skinless chicken breasts, cut into bite-sized pieces	
2 quarts gluten-free chicken broth	*2* Add the chicken broth, coconut milk, liquid aminos, brown sugar, red chili paste, mushrooms, jalapeño or serrano, ginger, and lime zest. Bring the mixture to a boil over high heat; then reduce the temperature to low and simmer for 10 minutes.
14.5-ounce can coconut milk	
2 tablespoons Bragg Liquid Aminos or coconut aminos	
1 tablespoon light brown sugar	*3* Stir in the lime juice, cilantro, and basil and serve. Season with salt to taste.
1 tablespoon red chili paste	
8 ounces white mushrooms, sliced	
1 small jalapeño or serrano pepper, thinly sliced	
1-inch piece fresh ginger, grated	
2 medium limes, zested and juiced	
1 cup chopped cilantro	
½ cup chopped basil	
Salt	

Per serving: Calories 419 (From Fat 252); Fat 28g (Saturated 21g); Cholesterol 63mg; Sodium 1,907mg; Carbohydrate 15g (Dietary Fiber 2g); Protein 29g.

Note: When slicing hot peppers, consider wearing gloves.

Tropical Kebabs with Coconut Curry Rice

Prep time: 25 min • **Cook time:** 25 min • **Yield:** 4 servings

Ingredients	Directions
1 pound boneless, skinless chicken breasts, cut into 1-inch pieces	*1* In a shallow mixing bowl, place the chicken, 1 tablespoon coconut milk, the zest of one lime, lime juice, pineapple juice, and liquid aminos. (**Tip:** Pour the pineapple juice from the bowl you put the cored pineapple in.) Allow the chicken to marinate on the counter for 20 minutes.
14.5-ounce can coconut milk, divided	
2 limes, zested and juiced (zest divided)	
1 tablespoon pineapple juice (from fresh pineapple)	*2* Meanwhile, in a 2-quart saucepan, bring the remaining coconut milk, the rest of the lime zest, the water, and the curry powder to a boil over high heat.
1 tablespoon Bragg Liquid Aminos or coconut aminos	
½ cup water	*3* Add the jasmine rice to the boiling coconut milk. Stir the mixture and bring it back to a boil. Cover the rice, reduce the heat to low, and allow the mixture to simmer for 25 minutes, or until all the liquid has been absorbed. Add the chopped cilantro and sliced almonds and then gently fluff the rice with a fork.
1 tablespoon curry powder	
1 cup jasmine rice	
½ cup chopped cilantro	
½ cup sliced almonds	*4* Heat a grill or grill pan over medium-high heat.
1 pineapple, peeled and cored, cut into bite-sized pieces	*5* Assemble the kebabs on skewers, alternating pineapple, bell pepper, onion, zucchini, and marinated chicken. Grill the kebabs for approximately 6 minutes on each side, or until the chicken is thoroughly cooked (165 degrees internal temperature). Serve the kebabs with the curried rice.
1 medium red bell pepper, cut into 1-inch squares	
1 medium sweet onion, peeled and cut into wedges	
2 medium zucchinis, sliced into ½-inch rounds	

Per serving: Calories 713 (From Fat 280); Fat 31g (Saturated 21g); Cholesterol 63mg; Sodium 247mg; Carbohydrate 81g (Dietary Fiber 8g); Protein 34g.

Vary It! Jasmine rice (Thai fragrant rice) is a variety of long-grain rice. Any rice (basmati, brown, and so on) can work in this recipe, as can a variety of vegetables (cauliflower, Brussels sprouts, eggplant, and the like).

Note: To cut down on preparation time, look for a cored and peeled pineapple in the refrigerator section of your grocery store.

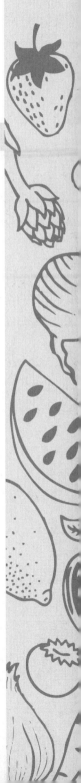

Southwestern Turkey Chili

Prep time: 15 min • **Cook time:** 50 min • **Yield:** 8 servings

Ingredients	*Directions*
1 tablespoon olive oil	*1* In a large stockpot or Dutch oven, heat the olive oil over medium-high heat. Add the ground turkey breast to the pot and cook until it's browned, about 10 minutes. Remove the turkey and set it aside.
2 pounds ground turkey breast	
1 medium onion, diced	
2 medium carrots, diced	*2* Add the onion, carrots, celery, red bell pepper, green bell pepper, and jalapeño to the stockpot. Sauté the vegetables for 10 minutes.
2 celery stalks, diced	
1 medium red bell pepper, diced	
1 medium green bell pepper, diced	*3* Return the cooked turkey to the stockpot and add the garlic, beef broth, diced tomatoes, tomato sauce, chili powder, pinto beans, and kidney beans. Bring the mixture to a boil over medium heat. Then reduce the heat to low, cover, and simmer for 30 minutes.
1 small jalapeño, minced	
4 cloves garlic, chopped	
1 quart gluten-free beef broth	
28-ounce can diced tomatoes	
14.5-ounce can tomato sauce	
¼ cup chili powder	
14.5-ounce can pinto beans, drained and rinsed	
14.5-ounce can kidney beans, drained and rinsed	

Per serving: Calories 304 (From Fat 39); Fat 4g (Saturated 1g); Cholesterol 77mg; Sodium 1,020mg; Carbohydrate 30g (Dietary Fiber 9g); Protein 37g.

Chapter 17

Savoring a Snack or Something Sweet

. . . .

. . . .

*W*hen you think of snacking, images of cookies, cakes, and sodas may come to mind. That type of snacking can send your blood glucose levels skyrocketing and cause your long-term energy to crash. But when you snack wisely on foods that provide sustenance, you help your body maintain an even blood glucose level, which is especially important for people with adrenal fatigue. Thus, smart snacking wins!

However, we understand that sometimes you want food just because it looks, smells, feels, and tastes good — those foods are more of an indulgence. In this chapter, you gain a greater knowledge of how to approach the urge to eat a snack or dessert. We help you pair foods and look toward food choices that can satisfy your cravings without sparking an insulin response. We also examine the smart way to eat for pleasure and show you how to approach something rich and decadent so that your snacks don't become snack attacks.

Here, we've brought both kinds of snacks together — the smart snacks and the little indulgences. You can decide for yourself whether you're truly hungry and which foods will satisfy the urge for a sweet nosh or a satiating snack.

Snacking with Low Glycemic Loads

The *glycemic index (GI)* is the measurement of how a particular carbohydrate food affects blood glucose, benchmarked against pure glucose. Snacks that have a low glycemic index are less apt to stimulate the adrenal hormones such as cortisol and to raise and then drop blood glucose levels.

The *glycemic load (GL)* takes into account the serving size of the carbohydrate food and its effect on blood glucose. Foods with both a low glycemic index and low glycemic load are less likely to cause hypoglycemia.

Portion size, fiber content, and food combinations all influence the glycemic load of a snack or meal. Smart snacks for people with adrenal fatigue combine protein with a little fat and carbohydrates, as in a handful of almonds with an apple or hummus with carrot sticks.

A lot of information in the media on what foods do to blood sugar is inaccurate, but we have excellent data on actual glycemic indexes as well as the glycemic loads of foods. These two factors played a key role in developing the snack and dessert recipes in this chapter.

You can find more information on the glycemic index and glycemic loads in *Glycemic Index Diet For Dummies,* by Meri Reffetto, RD; in *Glycemic Index Cookbook For Dummies,* by Meri Reffetto, RD, and Rosanne Rust, MS, RD, LDN; and in the articles at www.dummies.com. More technical information through the Linus Pauling Institute is at http://lpi.oregonstate.edu/infocenter/foods/grains/gigl.html.

Eating probiotic snacks

Probiotics, the good bacteria, have a mutually beneficial relationship with the human body (see Chapter 11 for details). They're responsible for the breakdown and absorption of many nutrients, they help keep your digestive tract clear to allow nutrient absorption, and they keep digestion moving to ensure excretion of waste. You can use snack time to get some probiotics into your diet. Here are some perfect probiotic snacks:

- Kimchi on rice crackers with a handful of nuts
- Sauerkraut and bites of roasted meat (pork or turkey)
- Kefir
- Greek yogurt and your favorite fruit

Eating for Pleasure: The Three-Bite Rule

Should you be snacking all day? Or eating six small meals throughout the day? The answer varies; in truth, it's more about tuning in to your body's cues of hunger and then taking in nourishment when you need it — before you find yourself feasting on foods that sound good but don't provide the sustenance your body needs. With the concept of mindful eating in mind (see Chapter 16), ask yourself these questions:

- ✔ Am I really hungry, or do I just have a desire to eat?
- ✔ If I'm hungry, does a piece of fruit sound good to me?

If a piece of fruit doesn't sound appealing, go back to the first question. You may be tuning in to your appetite rather than actual hunger cues. Simply speaking, *hunger* is the physiological need for food, and *appetite* is the desire for food.

Although it's easy to say you should eat only when you're hungry, that's hard to do. At times, you may just desire the texture of food or the comfort of having something to eat. In these instances, the Three-Bite Rule can help you enjoy a sweet or savory snack — and step away from it, too, feeling satisfied.

Here's how the Three-Bite Rule works. Try it out with a couple of 0.5-ounce pieces of chocolate (preferably high-quality, 65 percent cacao or greater). You'll take three bites of the first piece of chocolate, so be sure to pace yourself:

1. **Take a bite and focus only on the texture.**

   Describe the texture. Is it smooth? Crispy? Crunchy? Grainy? Silky?

2. **Take a second bite and focus only on the flavor.**

   Is it bitter? Sweet? Fruity? Tart? Salty? Rich? Smoky? Milky?

3. **For the last bite, pull both factors together. Focus on the texture *and* flavor.**

   How was the final bite? Could you say that you got the full chocolate experience within just three bites?

Now pop the second piece of chocolate into your mouth and eat it as fast as you can. How satisfying was that? Or rather, how *dissatisfying?*

The point of this exercise is to note how satisfied you can be with just three bites. If you tune in to each and every bite, it's easier to step away from the food. Try it. Start and finish each and every meal with such focus and see how your satisfaction increases with each bite!

The preceding exercise is based on research on eating mindfully. You can view more information at www.apa.org/monitor/2012/11/bite-chew.aspx.

I (coauthor Wendy Jo) once tried this activity using M&M mini bags with a group of children. I asked them to eat their first bag the way they normally would. The majority of the kids opened the bag and poured it into their mouths, taking maybe less than 3 seconds to inhale the M&Ms. Then I asked them to rate their satisfaction, and they all wanted more. Next, I asked them to tune in to their M&Ms as they ate them, following the principles of the Three-Bite Rule. Interestingly, many of the kids said the chocolate tasted waxy, and it was no longer their favorite candy. I'm sure I created some chocolate snobs in that class, and I consider that a job well done!

Afternoon Cinnamon Pumpkin Latte

Prep time: 3 min • **Cook time:** 3 min • **Yield:** 1 serving

Ingredients	Directions
1 fluid ounce (2 tablespoons) brewed espresso (instant or fresh)	**1** Put the espresso in a large coffee mug and set it aside.
1 cup almond milk **¼ cup canned pumpkin puree** **1 teaspoon honey** **½ teaspoon pumpkin pie spice**	**2** In a small saucepan, add the almond milk, pumpkin puree, honey, and pumpkin pie spice. Bring the mixture to a simmer over medium-high heat (about 3 minutes).
	3 Pour the heated milk mixture over the espresso, stir, and serve.

Per serving: Calories 108 (From Fat 26); Fat 3g (Saturated 0g); Cholesterol 0mg; Sodium 149mg; Carbohydrate 20g (Dietary Fiber 4g); Protein 3g.

Vary It! You can use coconut milk in place of the almond milk.

Note: An ounce of espresso contains about 30 milligrams of caffeine, similar to a cup of hot tea. If you're sensitive to caffeine, use decaffeinated espresso or chicory tea as an alternative.

Chocolate, Banana, and Almond Butter Smoothie

Prep time: 3 min • **Yield:** 1 serving

Ingredients	Directions
½ of a medium frozen banana	*1* Put the half banana, chocolate protein powder, almond butter, spinach, coconut milk, and ice in a blender. Blend at high speed for 3 minutes, or until the smoothie reaches your desired consistency. Serve the smoothie immediately.
1 to 2 scoops chocolate protein powder (egg white, whey, or pea protein powder)	
1 tablespoon almond butter (no salt or sugar added)	
1 cup spinach	
1 cup coconut milk	
Ice, as desired	

Per serving: Calories 218 (From Fat 56); Fat 6g (Saturated 4g); Cholesterol 0mg; Sodium 444mg; Carbohydrate 19g (Dietary Fiber 4g); Protein 24g.

Vary It! You can use kefir in place of the coconut milk. Also consider using kale or Swiss chard in place of spinach for increased nutritional value.

Spiced Coconut Hot Cocoa

Prep time: 5 min • **Cook time:** 5 min • **Yield:** 2 servings

Ingredients	Directions
2½ cups refrigerated or boxed coconut milk	**1** In a 2-quart saucepan, heat the coconut milk, honey, cocoa powder, cinnamon, ginger, cayenne pepper, and salt over medium-high heat, stirring constantly, until the spiced cocoa reaches a simmer.
2 tablespoons honey	
3 tablespoons cocoa powder	
⅛ teaspoon ground cinnamon	**2** Remove the spiced cocoa from the heat and stir in the vanilla extract. Serve immediately in two large mugs.
⅛ teaspoon ground ginger	
1 pinch cayenne pepper	
1 pinch salt	
¼ teaspoon vanilla extract	

Per serving: Calories 141 (From Fat 61); Fat 6g (Saturated 0g); Cholesterol 0mg; Sodium 91mg; Carbohydrate 25g (Dietary Fiber 4g); Protein 2g.

Pear, Walnut, Goat Cheese, and Honey Stacks

Prep time: 10 min • **Yield:** 4 servings

Ingredients	Directions
3 medium pears, cut into ⅛-inch thick slices	*1* Place the pear slices on a plate. Sprinkle goat cheese and walnuts over the pear slices.
3 ounces goat cheese, crumbled	
½ cup walnuts, chopped	*2* Drizzle the pears with honey and serve.
1 tablespoon honey	

Per serving: Calories 234 (From Fat 121); Fat 14g (Saturated 4g); Cholesterol 27mg; Sodium 103mg; Carbohydrate 26g (Dietary Fiber 6g); Protein 7g.

Greek Yogurt Spinach Dip

Prep time: 10 min • **Chill time:** 1 hr • **Yield:** 10 servings

Ingredients	Directions
3 cups plain Greek yogurt	**1** In a mixing bowl, stir together the yogurt, spinach, spinach dip or soup mix, onion, and red bell pepper.
12-ounce bag frozen spinach, defrosted and squeezed dry	
Half of a 1.4-ounce package Simply Organic Spinach Dip Mix or powdered vegetable soup mix	**2** Refrigerate the dip for at least 1 hour before serving to allow the flavors to meld. Serve with carrot and/or celery sticks.
½ red onion, finely chopped	
½ red bell pepper, seeded and finely chopped	
30 carrot or celery sticks	

Per serving: Calories 68 (From Fat 13); Fat 1g (Saturated 1g); Cholesterol 5mg; Sodium 232mg; Carbohydrate 7g (Dietary Fiber 1g); Protein 7g.

Vary It! You can use coconut yogurt, which uses coconut milk instead of dairy as the base, in place of the Greek yogurt. Or if you don't like carrots and celery, you can serve this delicious dip with a variety of other snacking vegetables, such as cucumbers, bell peppers, cauliflower, and broccoli florets.

Tip: If you're concerned about sodium in your diet, replace the mix with a salt-free seasoning blend. We suggest ¼ cup Mrs. Dash Onion & Herb Seasoning Blend.

Lentil Hummus

Prep time: 5 min • **Cook time:** 35 min • **Yield:** 8 servings

Ingredients	Directions
2 cups water	**1** In a small saucepan, bring the water and lentils to a boil over medium-high heat. Then reduce the heat to low and continue to cook, allowing the lentils to absorb the water (about 25 to 30 minutes).
1 cup brown lentils, rinsed and drained	
1 clove garlic	
½ medium lemon, juiced	**2** Add the cooked lentils to a food processor with the garlic clove, lemon juice, tahini, olive oil, and salt. Process the mixture into a smooth paste. Serve with vegetables of your choice.
2 tablespoons tahini (sesame paste)	
1 tablespoon olive oil	
¼ teaspoon salt	

Per serving: Calories 119 (From Fat 35); Fat 4g (Saturated 1g); Cholesterol 0mg; Sodium 76mg; Carbohydrate 15g (Dietary Fiber 6g); Protein 7g.

Vary It! Feel free to experiment with herbs and spices such as cayenne pepper, basil, or sun-dried tomatoes to change the flavor of the hummus and to kick up the antioxidant profile! You can also increase the amount of garlic if you like.

Antioxidant Spiced Nuts

Prep time: 5 min • **Cook time:** 25 min • **Yield:** 24 servings (¼ cup each)

Ingredients	Directions
1 tablespoon olive oil	*1* Preheat the oven to 350 degrees. Brush a baking sheet with olive oil.
2½ cups cashews	
1½ cups walnuts	*2* Combine the cashews, walnuts, pecans, almonds, maple syrup, brown sugar, orange juice, chipotle powder, and 2 tablespoons of rosemary in a large mixing bowl. Mix well and pour the nuts onto the baking sheet.
1½ cups pecan halves	
½ cup almonds	
⅓ cup maple syrup	
¼ cup brown sugar	*3* Spread the nuts into a single layer and roast them for 25 minutes. Stir the mixture with a spatula twice during the roasting time (about every 8 minutes or so).
3 tablespoons orange juice	
2 tablespoons chipotle chile powder	*4* Remove the nuts from the oven and sprinkle them with salt and the remaining 2 tablespoons of rosemary. Toss the nuts well.
4 tablespoons minced fresh rosemary, divided	
1 teaspoon kosher salt	*5* As the nuts cool, stir them occasionally to prevent sticking. After the nuts have cooled, store them in an airtight container.

Per serving: Calories 195 (From Fat 141); Fat 16g (Saturated 2g); Cholesterol 0mg; Sodium 95mg; Carbohydrate 12g (Dietary Fiber 2g); Protein 7g.

Chi-Chi-Chi Chia Pudding

Prep time: 3 min • **Chill time:** 4 hr • **Yield:** 2 servings

Ingredients	Directions
¼ cup chia seeds	*1* In a glass jar, mix the chia seeds, coconut milk, honey, and cherries. Shake well.
1 cup refrigerated or boxed coconut milk	
2 tablespoons honey	*2* Seal the jar with a lid and refrigerate the pudding for 4 hours or overnight. The chia seeds will plump up, making the pudding look similar to tapioca pudding.
½ cup dried tart cherries	
¼ teaspoon vanilla or almond extract	

Per serving: Calories 304 (From Fat 78); Fat 9g (Saturated 3g); Cholesterol 0mg; Sodium 12mg; Carbohydrate 52g (Dietary Fiber 9g); Protein 5g.

Vary It! You can use almond or rice milk in place of the coconut milk. You can also change the flavor by trying a variety of dried or fresh fruits. For a decadent treat, use chocolate almond milk and bananas.

A power-packed seed

Looking for a nutrient-rich and healthy snack to eat on the go? Chia seeds offer a great way to get some essential nutrients quickly. Chia seeds, from the plant *Salvia hispanica*, are good sources of omega-3 fatty acids, phosphorus, manganese, calcium, potassium, and sodium. That's a lot of nutrients you can sprinkle on just about anything! An ounce of dried chia seeds contains 4 grams of protein, 9 grams of fat, and 11 grams of fiber.

Unlike flaxseed, chia seeds can be stored for long periods without becoming rancid, and they don't require grinding. Whole flaxseed is tough to digest and simply doesn't agree with everyone, so instead, give chia a try!

Greek Yogurt Key Lime Pie

Prep time: 10 min • **Cook time:** 15 min • **Chill time:** 1 hr • **Yield:** 8 servings

Ingredients	*Directions*
2½ cups gluten-free gingersnap cookies	*1* Preheat the oven to 350 degrees.
6 tablespoons vegan butter spread, butter, or coconut oil	*2* In a food processor, blend the gingersnap cookies into fine crumbs.
¾ cup key lime juice (from about 7 key limes)	*3* Add slices of cold butter spread to the crumbs and pulse until combined. Pour the crumbs into a 9-inch pie pan and press down with your fingertips to form the crust.
Two 14-ounce cans sweetened condensed milk	
1 cup plain Greek yogurt (whole or 2% fat)	*4* Bake the crust for 8 minutes. Remove it from the oven and chill it while you prepare the filling.
	5 Whisk together the key lime juice, sweetened condensed milk, and Greek yogurt. Pour the filling into the crust.
	6 Bake the pie for 12 to 15 minutes. Chill the pie in the refrigerator for at least 1 hour prior to slicing.

Per serving: Calories 532 (From Fat 157); Fat 18g (Saturated 6g); Cholesterol 35mg; Sodium 338mg; Carbohydrate 86g (Dietary Fiber 3g); Protein 13g.

Tip: Add 1 tablespoon lime zest to the filling for an extra dose of lime.

Vary It! Bake the pie in individual portions using custard cups, ramekins, or small Mason jars. Reduce the baking time for single servings, cooking the crust for only 3 to 4 minutes and the pies for 8 to 10 minutes. Shake the custards; if they seem firm, they're ready to be pulled from the oven.

Almond and Apricot Truffles

Prep time: 20 min • **Cook time:** 5 min • **Chill time:** 30 min • **Yield:** 30 servings

Ingredients	Directions
1⅓ cup raw, unsalted almonds	**1** Toast the almonds in a skillet over medium heat. Stirring frequently, heat the nuts until they're fragrant, about 5 minutes.
1 cup dried apricots	
3 tablespoons honey	**2** Put the almonds and apricots in a food processor and pulse for 30 seconds. Add the honey, cocoa powder, vanilla, and salt to the almond mixture and process for 1 minute. Slowly add enough water to the almond mixture, pulsing the mixture until a dough forms.
½ cup cocoa powder	
2 teaspoon vanilla extract	
⅛ teaspoon salt	
1 tablespoon water	**3** Scoop out 1 tablespoon of the mixture and form it into a ball using your hands. Repeat until you've shaped all the mixture.
	4 Refrigerate the truffles for at least 30 minutes before serving.

Per serving: Calories 59 (From Fat 30); Fat 3g (Saturated 0g); Cholesterol 0mg; Sodium 11mg; Carbohydrate 7g (Dietary Fiber 2g); Protein 2g.

Vary It! Replace ⅓ cup almonds with pistachios.

Chocolate Coconut Custard with Almonds

Prep time: 10 min • **Cook time:** 12 min • **Chill time:** 8 hr • **Yield:** 8 servings

Ingredients	Directions
½ **gallon boxed or refrigerated coconut milk**	*1* In a 6-quart saucepan over medium heat, whisk together the coconut milk, maple syrup, egg yolks, gelatin, and cocoa powder. Cook the custard, whisking continuously, until it's slightly thickened and begins to simmer, about 8 to 12 minutes.
½ **cup maple syrup**	
3 **egg yolks, beaten**	
Two 0.25-ounce envelopes unflavored gelatin	*2* Remove the saucepan from the heat and pour the custard mixture into a large glass bowl. Stir in the vanilla extract. Cover the bowl with plastic wrap, with the plastic wrap directly touching the custard to prevent a skin from forming on the surface. Refrigerate the custard for at least 8 hours before serving; the custard will thicken as it chills.
3 **tablespoons cocoa powder**	
1 **teaspoon vanilla extract**	
2 **cups almonds**	
	3 In a food processor, pulse the almonds for 4 minutes, or until they resemble a fine breadcrumb. Divide the custard among eight custard cups or small wide-mouthed mason jars, sprinkle with almond crumbs, and serve.

Per serving: Calories 335 (From Fat 217); Fat 24g (Saturated 6g); Cholesterol 69mg; Sodium 25mg; Carbohydrate 25g (Dietary Fiber 6g); Protein 11g.

Vary It! You can use honey in place of the maple syrup.

Tip: Don't have custard cups? Use a muffin pan! Line your muffin pan with foil cupcake liners. The liners are smaller, so you'll likely get 12 servings instead.

Tart Cherry Granola

Prep time: 10 min • **Cook time:** 35 min • **Yield:** 12 servings

Ingredients	Directions
2 cups gluten-free oats	**1** Preheat the oven to 300 degrees. Line a 9-x-13-inch baking pan with parchment paper.
1 cup unsweetened coconut	
¼ cup chia seeds	**2** In a large bowl, mix together the oats, coconut, chia seeds, and puffed millet.
1 cup puffed millet	
¼ cup vegan butter spread or butter	**3** In a heavy 2-quart saucepan, heat the butter spread, honey, and brown sugar over medium-high heat until the mixture comes to a boil. Remove the saucepan from the heat and stir in the vanilla extract.
⅔ cup honey	
¼ cup packed brown sugar	
1 teaspoon vanilla extract	
1 cup dried tart cherries	**4** Pour the hot mixture over the oat/coconut/millet mixture. Then stir in the dried cherries and salt. Press the mixture into the baking pan.
¼ teaspoon salt	
	5 Bake the granola for 25 to 35 minutes, or until it's golden brown, stirring the mixture every 10 minutes.
	6 Allow the mixture to cool for at least 3 hours before serving. Store the granola in an airtight container at room temperature for 1 week or in the freezer for up to 3 months.

Per serving: Calories 267 (From Fat 74); Fat 8g (Saturated 5g); Cholesterol 0mg; Sodium 93mg; Carbohydrate 44g (Dietary Fiber 4g); Protein 5g.

Note: Millet is a popular gluten-free seed gaining popularity in recipes due to its nutrient density and mild taste.

Part V
The Part of Tens

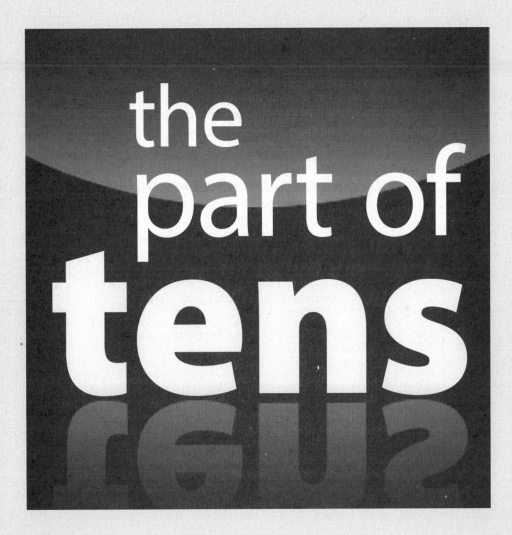

Check out an additional Part of Tens list about foods that boost adrenal function at www.dummies.com/extras/adrenalfatigue.

In this part...

✔ Review ten great ways to combat depression in adrenal fatigue patients. You can enjoy moderate exercise, yoga, vitamins and other nutrients, and natural supplements.

✔ Discover ten effective supplements for boosting your immune system. Strengthening your immune system is key to helping your adrenal glands overcome adrenal fatigue. An optimized immune system is better able to fight off infections and handle inflammation, dramatically decreasing adrenal gland stress.

✔ Use ten simple tricks to optimize the function of your organs and systems. A problem with one organ can negatively affect other organs, including your adrenal glands.

Chapter 18

More Than Ten Ways to Help Beat Depression in Adrenal Fatigue

· ·

In This Chapter

▶ Improving your mood with exercise, yoga, and aromatherapy

▶ Including nutrients, vitamins, and natural supplements in your routine

▶ Balancing your pH

▶ Trying a detox program

· ·

Depression is a significant symptom of adrenal fatigue (as you find out in Chapter 4). This chapter discusses several ways to try to beat depression, including moderate exercise, yoga, nutrients, and natural supplements. *Note:* A deficiency in essential nutrients can contribute to the development of depression. As health professionals, we first and foremost recommend improving your diet, as we discuss in Chapter 8 and Part IV. To fully overcome depression in the setting of adrenal fatigue, however, additional supplements, including those you read about in this chapter, may be necessary.

Depression can be very isolating. It's important to reach out to a family member, significant other, or friend to help you get better. Sometimes, just talking can be a great stress-reliever that improves your mood. Many causes of depression may be related to adrenal fatigue, so do all you can to treat adrenal fatigue, fight the depression, and seek the help of a mental health professional if needed.

Improving Mood with Exercise

Exercise is one of the best ways to beat depression. In addition to relieving stress and building strength and stamina, exercise improves and stabilizes your mood. The thinking is that exercise changes neurotransmitters and other brain factors.

Is one type of exercise better than another? Well, a study in the *American Journal of Preventive Nutrition* in 2005 reported that to improve mood, aerobic exercise should be mildly vigorous in intensity. In the study, very light exercise didn't appear to have a significant effect on reducing symptoms of depression.

This doesn't mean that you shouldn't do muscle resistance training. A study in the *Journal of Strength and Conditioning Research* in 2010 evaluated the effects of a muscle resistance training program for individuals who were diagnosed with depression and who also had risk factors for obesity and Type II diabetes mellitus. The researchers concluded that resistance training, done on a moderate to high level of intensity, improved mood (and of course, the exercise helps obesity and diabetes, too).

The take-home message seems to be this: Moderate-intensity exercise performed on a regular basis is beneficial in treating depression. That being said, everyone has to start somewhere. If you have fibromyalgia, you don't want to go hog wild in intensity when you first start an exercise program. You may not be able to exercise much at first, or you may actually feel worse afterward. Building up your exercise program slowly and carefully over time can be very beneficial in reducing the symptoms of depression.

Please refer to Chapter 12 for more information on exercise and consult your healthcare provider concerning the type, intensity, and frequency of your exercise regimen.

Practicing Yoga

Studies have shown that yoga can help in treating depression. It can also increase muscle flexibility, reduce pain, and improve overall *functional status* (a person's ability to function independently on his or her own and success-fully perform the activities of daily living).

A study published in *Complementary Therapies in Medicine* in June 2012 evaluated 80 patients with low back pain, randomizing them into either a yoga regimen or a physical exercise regimen. Although pain and symptoms of depression decreased in both groups, the authors of the study concluded that yoga was more effective than more-vigorous exercise.

Yoga has other health benefits, too (see Chapter 12). Consider adding yoga to your daily regimen to help improve your mood, flexibility, and sense of well-being.

Sniffing Your Way to a Better Mood

Aromatherapy can be a great way to not only improve your mood but also help you get a good night's sleep. Improving sleep can do wonders to alleviate symptoms of depression.

Studies have shown that lavender oil in particular can improve sleep and reduce depression. One 2006 study in the Korean journal *Taehan Kanho Hakhoe Chi* evaluated more than 40 college-age women who were exposed to a lavender fragrance overnight while sleeping. Compared to a placebo group, the group exposed to the lavender fragrance reported reduced symptoms of depression and improved sleep. The nose knows, and the use of essential oils like lavender can make you feel like a new person. (The oils smell nice, too!)

Aromatherapy can be useful in helping you overcome depression. Here are a couple of ways that coauthor Rich's patients have used lavender oil at night to help them sleep:

✔ Add two or three drops of lavender oil to a cotton ball. Put the cotton ball next to you on your pillow while you're sleeping.

✔ Rub a couple of drops of lavender oil on each temple before going to sleep.

A great reference guide for understanding the basics of aromatherapy is *Aromatherapy For Dummies,* by Kathi Keville (published by Wiley).

Opting for Omega-3s

Several studies in the *Journal of Clinical Psychiatry* in 2011 and 2013 demonstrated that major depression involves a deficiency in omega-3 polyunsaturated fatty acids. Researchers identified low levels of DHA (docosahexaenoic acid) and EPA (eicosapentaenoic acid) as contributors to depression; supplementation of omega-3 fatty acids can help normalize EPA and DHA levels.

The *Journal of Clinical Psychiatry* in 2011 reviewed more than 15 clinical trials with more than 900 participants, examining the effects of omega-3 fatty acid supplementation. The authors concluded that supplementation with omega-3 fish oil was effective in treating depression. They specifically recommended that the amount of EPA in the omega-3 fish oil (compared to the amount of DHA) be more than 60 percent of the total formulation.

The Western or standard American diet contains processed foods that are high in omega-6 fatty acids and low in omega-3s. This ratio only perpetuates inflammation and therefore can contribute to depression. Omega-6 fatty acids are pro-inflammatory and bad for your health; omega-3 fatty acids are beneficial for your health. The goal is to have a higher level of omega-3s and a lower level of omega-6s in your diet.

A recommended starting dose of omega-3 fish oil is 2 grams a day, taken with food, usually in divided doses. Eating foods high in omega-3s, such as salmon, can certainly help, too, but the treatment of depression may require higher doses that what you can get from food.

Omega-3 fish oil supplements are generally safe to take on your own. As with all supplements, speak with your healthcare practitioner if you decide to increase your dose; it's always best to increase the dose gradually.

Various forms of dementia, including Alzheimer's dementia, have shown improvement with omega-3 supplementation. The symptoms of brain fog, including confusion and loss of short-term memory, can also be improved by omega-3 supplementation.

Seeking Out SAM-e

S-adenosyl-L-methionine (SAM-e) is a very well-researched supplement for treating depression. SAM-e is found in every living cell in the body; the body creates it from *methionine,* which is a naturally occurring amino acid, and *ATP (adenosine triphosphate),* the coenzyme your cells use to mobilize energy efficiently. SAM-e enables the many chemical processes that occur in cells. Physiologically, it does so by donating a methyl group (a process called *methylation*).

Several studies show that supplementing with SAM-e helps in the treatment of depression. One study in the *American Journal of Psychiatry* in 2010 showed that SAM-e helped alleviate the symptoms of depression in patients who didn't respond to medication therapy. The mechanism by which SAM-e works to treat depression isn't fully known, but it may have to do with increasing the levels of serotonin and other brain hormones.

You should take SAM-e only under the watchful eye of your healthcare practitioner. You usually take it orally, although it can be given intravenously or as an intramuscular injection. Commonly, lower doses of SAM-e are preferred to start with; then your healthcare provider slowly increases the dose as needed. A typical starting dose is a 200-milligram capsule taken daily in the morning with food.

Several studies have shown that SAM-e also has positive and protective effects on liver function.

Taking Your B Vitamins

Certain vitamin deficiencies may predispose you to developing depression. One of them is a vitamin B_{12} deficiency. A study in the *American Journal of Psychiatry* in 2000 evaluated levels of B_{12}, folate (another B vitamin), and their metabolites in more than 700 women aged 65 and older who had a physical disability. They found that women who had metabolically low vitamin B_{12} levels were at a significant risk of developing severe depression, even if their blood levels were low normal.

The phrase *metabolically low* suggests that measuring B_{12} levels in the blood (as most healthcare professionals routinely do) may not be enough to document B_{12} deficiency. When comparing the individuals with depression to those without it, the researchers found no statistically significant differences in the B_{12} levels in the blood. When methylmalonic acid levels were measured, however, the individuals who were depressed demonstrated high levels of this *metabolite* (a breakdown product of the vitamin as it's processed by the body). It's the activity level of B_{12}, not just the blood level, that's important for your health. Nonetheless, supplementing with vitamin B_{12} is important for maintaining optimal blood levels.

Low vitamin B_6 levels also seem to be associated with increased risk of developing depression. In a study from the journal *Psychotherapy and Psychosomatics* in 2004, the authors noted that in an evaluation of 18 individuals who were diagnosed with clinical depression, the level of pyridoxal phosphate (an active form of B_6) was low in the blood. In another 2004 study in the same journal, 140 individuals were evaluated for symptoms of depression. Approximately 13 percent of the respondents fulfilled criteria for depression. Compared to the other respondents, the depressed group had lower blood levels of pyridoxal phosphate. The results of these two studies suggest that low vitamin B_6 levels are associated with the development of depression; therefore, supplementation with vitamin B_6 may help in treating depression.

A good starting dose for vitamin B_6 is 50 milligrams a day, and a good starting dose for vitamin B_{12} is 250 micrograms a day. Stomach acid can break down vitamin B_{12}, rendering it ineffective, so a great way to take B_{12} is under the tongue (sublingually) to maximize its absorption. Both vitamins can be taken in the morning. Vitamin B_6 should be taken with food. Please refer to Chapter 11 for more information on vitamin B_6 and B_{12} supplementation.

Visiting Vitamin D

Vitamin D deficiency has been found to contribute to depression. In one study published in the *Journal of Clinical Psychopharmacology* in 2013, more than 40 patients were diagnosed with depression and low vitamin D levels. Replacement with high doses of vitamin D showed an improvement in depressive symptoms. Another study in the journal *Clinical Rheumatology* in 2007 demonstrated that vitamin D supplementation can help ameliorate depression symptoms in someone with fibromyalgia syndrome (FMS). This finding is important because FMS is so closely related to adrenal fatigue (see Chapter 7 for details).

The ways in which low vitamin D_3 levels contribute to the development of depression are still being studied. Vitamin D_3 is important for many body processes, and it likely plays a role in brain chemistry as well. The skin can produce vitamin D_3 with adequate sunlight, so in winter, the body's levels of vitamin D_3 tend to be at their lowest; seasonal affective disorder (a type of depression) occurs with increased frequency.

For more information on vitamin D_3 supplementation, please refer to Chapter 11.

Eliminating Yeast

There's a significant connection between intestinal health and the development of depression. One of the biggest contributors to depression is the overgrowth of *Candida,* a genus of yeast. Yeast overgrowth affects the ability of the intestine to absorb micronutrients. These nutritional deficiencies likely contribute to depression by altering brain chemistry.

Eliminating the yeast from your intestine can be one way to improve your mood. Add one or more of the following to your supplement regimen to help treat *Candida* overgrowth:

- Olive leaf extract
- Garlic
- Oil of oregano

Please refer to Chapter 11 for info on treating *Candida* overgrowth. Talk with your healthcare practitioner before implementing an anti-*Candida* regimen, because dosing will vary from person to person.

Besides eliminating yeast overgrowth, you can do other things to promote intestinal health. Using probiotics helps normalize the intestinal flora, which is integral in treating depression. Often, eliminating *Candida* overgrowth and taking probiotics happen in tandem. (See Chapter 11 for details on probiotics.)

Taking St. John's Wort

One of the most widely used natural treatments for depression is St. John's wort *(Hypericum perforatum)*. Studies have shown this herb to be very effective. Its mode of action is similar to that of prescription antidepressant medications, including tricyclic antidepressants. In the journal *Brain Research* in 1999, researchers proposed that St. John's wort affects the way that brain cells handle serotonin and norepinephrine.

St. John's wort can interact with other medications. This herb is called an *enzymatic inducer,* which means that it can speed up the liver's processing (metabolizing) of other medications. Medications may be eliminated from your body faster than they should be. Review all your medications with your healthcare practitioner. If you're taking St. John's wort, the doses of some of your medications may need adjustment, and levels of medications that require monitoring in the blood need to be monitored more frequently. Significant medication classes whose levels can be affected by St. John's wort include the following:

- ✔ Transplant-related medications, including cyclosporine and tacrolimus
- ✔ HIV-related medications
- ✔ Anti-cancer medications
- ✔ Warfarin (Coumadin)

Using St. John's wort isn't a good idea if you're taking prescription medications for the treatment of depression, including tricyclic antidepressants and selective serotonin reuptake inhibitors (SSRIs), such as sertraline (Zoloft) and fluoxetine (Prozac). St. John's wort can have really bad and potentially fatal reactions with these meds.

The usual starting dose of St. John's wort is 300 milligrams taken twice a day. Because this herb can interact with so many prescription medications, consult your healthcare provider before you begin to take St. John's wort.

Getting Back to Basics (pH)

Acidity isn't just at the heart of inflammation; it's also central to developing depression. A pH less than 7.0 is acidic, and a pH greater than 7.0 is basic (also called *alkaline*). One of the best things you can do for yourself in the morning is to alkalinize your pH, as measured in your urine. You'll find that as your urine becomes more alkaline, your mood dramatically improves.

Here are a few ways you can alkalinize your morning pH (people often use more than one of the following therapies):

✔ Add lemon to a regular glass of water. The body converts the lemon to citrate, which can make the urine more alkaline.

✔ Consume alkalinized water (see Chapter 11). You can purchase this water at your health food store, or you can make it yourself.

✔ Juice with alkaline-based fruits (including apples, berries, and pomegranate) and vegetables (such as eggplant, kale, and broccoli).

Detoxing Your Way Out of Depression

Every day you're exposed to toxins in the air, water, and food. You may encounter heavy metals, including lead and cadmium. And don't forget chemicals in detergents, cosmetics, insecticides, and pollutants. Even medications have levels of toxicity. Many of the artificial additives in your food can be toxic to your body as well.

Toxic substances can be a big contributor to depression, so you may want to consider a detox program. Detoxification involves a controlled elimination of toxic substances from the body. Most detox programs involve severely restricting your intake of toxic foods and liquids as well as taking a type of product that eliminates the toxins from your body, usually through your stool or urine. For example, many kidney-based detoxification programs use a substance called a *chelating agent*, which takes the toxins from the body and eliminates them via the urine. In a *sweat detox*, the toxins are expelled through the skin.

Supplementation with antioxidants, alkaline water, and nutrients is vital to prevent dehydration. It also helps ensure that your body and especially your adrenal glands get the nutrients they need.

Here are several important points to keep in mind when you're beginning a detox program:

- ✔ Consult with your healthcare practitioner before you start any detox program.

- ✔ A slow, ongoing detox program is safer and more beneficial than a quick detoxification. I (coauthor Rich) prefer a program that lasts 3 to 4 weeks at the bare minimum.

- ✔ With any type of detox program, you may feel worse before you feel better. That's why it's important to begin slowly.

- ✔ In the beginning, your healthcare provider should closely monitor your electrolytes, liver function, trace mineral status, and kidney function on a weekly basis. Without close monitoring in any detox program, you may be at risk for electrolyte imbalances, nutrient deficiencies, and dehydration.

- ✔ Keep a diary of what occurred each day, what you ate, your weight, and your blood pressure and pulse. This record-keeping is vital, especially if you're attempting a detox program in the advanced stages of adrenal fatigue.

Excellent references about detox programs include *Detox For Dummies,* by Dr. Caroline Shreeve, and *Detox Diets For Dummies,* by Dr. Gerald Don Wootan, DO, M.Ed., and M. Brittain Phillips (both published by Wiley).

Chapter 19

More Than Ten Supplements for Your Immune System

. . . .

In This Chapter

▶ Boosting your gut with probiotics, olive leaf extract, astragalus, and glutamine

▶ Supplementing with essential fats

▶ Protecting the brain, liver, and heart

. . . .

*O*ne of the most significant symptoms of adrenal fatigue is recurrent infections. For example, you may have repeated bouts of upper respiratory tract infections or bronchitis that you just can't seem to shake. That's likely due to a stressed-out immune system.

If you have adrenal fatigue, strengthening your immune system is important. Many of the supplements you read about in this chapter not only help you maintain a healthy immune system but also provide your immune system with a boost when it needs one. (Check out Chapter 11 for details on many of these supplements.)

Always consult your healthcare provider before taking any supplements. You may be able to obtain the supplements from your healthcare provider, or he or she may prescribe a specific type and dosage that you can get at your local health food store. Not all supplements are created equal, so if you're confused as to which brands are the best or a good buy, look to ConsumerLab.com (www.consumerlab.com). This independent watchdog organization ensures that what companies say about their products is true.

Use supplements to supplement your diet, not replace it! Although many people may try to convince you that the only way to heal is with supplements, focus on food and healthy habits first. Cleaning up your diet will set you on a track for long-term health and healing. Also make sure you aren't oversupplementing. If you're eating fortified foods, using boosted shakes, and taking vitamin complexes, you may find yourself taking in too much.

Taking Your Daily Probiotic

The intestine is filled with trillions of organisms that make up the *microflora* (also known as *microbiota* or *gut bugs*). Research shows that these creatures are vital for maintaining the body's immune response (see Chapter 8). A study from the journal *Nature* in 2013 suggests that your body's immune system may be able to recognize the good intestinal flora versus the bad intestinal flora. Having more of the bad flora compared to the good flora may send a signal to the body's immune system that sets it off. This explanation is likely an over-simplification, but several studies have demonstrated the importance of the intestinal ecosystem to regulating the immune system and inflammation.

You can increase the good flora in your intestine by taking a *probiotic,* which is a dose of live microorganisms. Many studies demonstrate the role of probiotics in treating chronic illness, suppressing inflammation, and helping many health conditions, including allergies and asthma.

Taking a probiotic once a day is good, but it may not be enough for most people. Many formulations allow you to take probiotic supplements up to three times a day.

Look for probiotic supplements in the refrigerated section of your health food store; probiotics are living things that survive best in cool temperatures. Don't just stop at one strain of bacteria, either! Look for a probiotic that has five to ten strains of bacteria, because science is still sorting out what each of these bugs does to boost your health.

When you think about probiotics, don't forget prebiotics (see Chapter 11). Probiotics and prebiotics pack a nice one-two punch!

Giving kids probiotics

Probiotics aren't just for adults. Consider starting your kids on probiotic supplements or adding a daily dose of fermented foods such as kefir or yogurt to their diets. A healthy immune system can pay huge dividends when the child reaches adulthood (and you'll save money, too, because the kid won't go to the doc as often).

In one study from the *British Journal of Nutrition* released in 2012, children were given a supplement that contained a fruit and vegetable concentrate, omega-3 fish oil, and probiotics; another group of children received a placebo. The authors concluded that the supplement that contained the probiotics decreased the use of medication and improved lung function.

Extending an Olive Branch: Olive Leaf Extract

Olive leaf extract is a wonderful antioxidant that has many properties, one of which is to enhance the immune system. It increases the immune system's ability to fight off infections, especially really bad viral infections. Did you know that olive leaf extract is effective against the flu? It's also a natural antibacterial and antifungal agent. As you read in Chapter 11, it can help in treating intestinal dysbiosis by helping eradicate *Candida* overgrowth in the gut.

In addition, olive leaf extract can lower blood pressure. One article from the journal *Phytomedicine* in 2011 found that doses of 500 milligrams of olive leaf extract twice a day had an effect that was similar to an equivalent dose of captopril, a prescription medication used to treat high blood pressure.

If you have advanced adrenal fatigue, speak with your healthcare practitioner concerning the optimal dose you should be on to reduce the risk of developing low blood pressure.

I (coauthor Rich) generally recommend beginning at a dose of 500 milligrams once a day. I prefer the capsules because they let you take an exact dose that can be adjusted. I ask that the patient monitor his or her blood pressure daily, and I normally assess how the patient is doing after 2 or more weeks.

Because olive leaf extract is a natural antibiotic, your healthcare practitioner may advise you to take a probiotic with it.

Supplementing with Vitamin D

Vitamin D should be a cornerstone of any health program. This vitamin is an important catalyst that helps your immune system mount an effective response to both bacterial and viral infections. Low levels of vitamin D_3 are associated with an increased risk of developing autoimmune diseases, such as lupus.

The most common dose of a vitamin D supplement is 1,000 international units (IU) of vitamin D_3 a day. It comes in softgels. This vitamin is fat-soluble, so your body absorbs it better when you take it with food. Your healthcare provider should routinely measure your vitamin D levels to help adjust your dose for maximum benefit.

Sunlight allows your body to make vitamin D. Head outside without sunblock for at least 15 minutes each day. Even people who live in sunny climates may still have low levels of vitamin D; you've got to *be* in the sun to get the benefit from the sun.

Opting for a Good Source of Omega-3s

Omega-3 fatty acids are the essential fats found in fatty fish, nuts, olives, and seeds. Omega-3s are directly linked to brain health, immunity, and reduced inflammation. A study in the journal *Immunity* in 2013 demonstrated that omega-3 fatty acids decrease the production of proteins that increase inflammation and rev up the immune system. Best that you get your share!

Omega-3s are commonly added to foods; however, the best way to get enough is through supplementing or through eating a diet naturally rich in omega-3s. When you look for a good omega-3 supplement, be sure to note the serving size (amount per tablet) and the quantity of eicosapentaenoic acid (EPA) and docosahexaenoic acid (DHA). Coauthor Wendy Jo recommends getting in a healthy dose of EPA and DHA equaling 2,000 milligrams per day.

To avoid getting the infamous fish burps, store your omega-3 supplements in the refrigerator. This protects the oils from going rancid. It's best to shop for the supplements in the refrigerated section of your local health food store as well.

Cod liver oil is an excellent way to take in both omega 3s and vitamin D in one. Your local health food store may even carry citrus-flavored oils to help you shoot it down the hatch.

Assessing the Awesome Astragalus

If you have a problem with recurrent allergies, consider using astragalus. *Astragalus* is an herb that has a beneficial effect on intestinal health, enhancing digestion and nutrient absorption. In addition, it's a great natural booster of your immune system. It can actually increase the number of immune cells to help your body fight off infection. To top it off, astragalus can also boost the function of the adrenal glands.

In the *Journal of Animal Science* in 2005, investigators used an animal-based study to evaluate the effects of astragalus supplementation on adrenal gland and immune system function. The animals were given a lipopolysaccharide, a substance that in humans is produced by bacteria that can cause a really bad infection in the blood. The authors noted that compared to the animals that didn't receive the astragalus, the treated group had higher levels of cortisol and glucose. The treated group also had a better immune response.

Although astragalus can be taken in different forms, I (coauthor Rich) prefer a capsule of astragalus root or extract because it's easy to take. Begin at 500 milligrams daily and take it with food. Most healthcare practitioners recommend doses of 500 to 1,000 milligrams a day.

Seeing Vitamin C

Talking about your immune system health without mentioning vitamin C would be impossible. This vitamin is known not only for having antioxidant properties but also for boosting the immune system. For example, ingesting vitamin C can help you fight off the flu during flu season.

An article from the *Annals of Nutrition and Metabolism* in 2006 reviewed the many benefits of vitamin C. It boosts the immune system's ability to eradicate infections by increasing the activity of certain aspects of the immune system, including the natural killer cells and lymphocytes. Don't forget that your adrenal glands need vitamin C as well; they soak up vitamin C like a sponge!

One of the best forms of vitamin C is the ester form; it is better absorbed and stays in the body for a longer period of time. I (coauthor Rich) recommend that everyone take at least 1,000 milligrams of vitamin C a day. Speak with your healthcare practitioner about increasing your dose, and refer to Chapter 11 for more information on vitamin C supplementation.

Beefing Up Your Immune Health with Beta-Glucans

Beta-glucans are immune-enhancing substances naturally found in yeast and certain grains, such as rye and wheat. They improve the communication between different aspects of your immune system. Be aware that your immune system involves a complex signaling pathway, with messages about recognizing foreign bacteria and viruses and mounting the body's immune response against them. You want the actors in your immune system talking to one another!

Beta-glucans are extracted from yeast and purified so you get the benefits of the beta-glucans but none of the problems with fungal overgrowth. In fact, beta-glucans can help in dealing with *Candida.*

I (coauthor Rich) prefer the capsule form of beta-glucans. There are many excellent name brands of beta-glucans, but be aware that beta-glucans made by different companies have different dosage formulations. Talk with your healthcare practitioner about whether beta-glucan supplementation may be appropriate for you. I commonly recommend taking one to two capsules a day on an empty stomach. You can take beta-glucans first thing in the morning.

Getting Tough with Turmeric

Turmeric is an antioxidant with anti-inflammatory properties. Not only does it benefit the adrenal glands, but it's also important for strengthening your immune system. Here are some of the benefits of turmeric:

- **Reducing inflammation:** Turmeric reduces the activity of certain inflammation pathways in the body. The active component of turmeric, *curcumin,* has been shown to reduce inflammation in many chronic illnesses.

- **Improving the immune system:** An article from the journal *Cellular Immunology* in 2012 suggests that turmeric enhances the ability of your immune system to fight off infections.

- **Protecting the heart and delaying diabetes:** Turmeric can help protect the heart from the effects of oxidative stress and inflammation. A few research studies have shown that turmeric delays the effects of insulin resistance, in turn delaying the development of diabetes. Diabetes is a risk factor for the development of heart disease.

- **Improving liver health:** A study in the journal *Phytomedicine* in 2012 used an animal model to explore the anti-inflammatory effects of curcumin. The study demonstrated that turmeric may bolster liver health by inhibiting oxidative stress and the resulting damage to the cells that occurs.

Although you commonly see turmeric as a ground spice, you can find fresh turmeric root in most specialty markets. The appearance is similar to gingerroot, but the inside of the turmeric root is bright orange. Turmeric is used extensively in South Asian cooking, particularly in India, Indonesia, and Vietnam.

Taking turmeric can be as simple as buying the powdered form of the spice and putting a little on each meal. It can make a mean salad even tastier or add flavor and color to your favorite grain side dish! However, probably the most convenient way to take turmeric is the capsule form. I (coauthor Rich) recommend taking a 400-milligram capsule daily in the morning. You can take it on an empty stomach.

Looking at L-lysine

L-lysine is an amino acid that isn't made by the human body, so you need to get it from other sources. It has several functions:

- ✔ It inhibits the replication of viruses, especially the herpes virus.
- ✔ It may help in treating diabetes by helping lower blood glucose levels.
- ✔ It's an important building block for cartilage, bones, and joints.

I (coauthor Rich) recommend dosages of 500 milligrams a day. Here are a couple of ways you can take L-lysine:

- ✔ I take a pill form of lysine that's made with proline (another amino acid) on a daily basis.
- ✔ If you're not a pill person, try a protein powder that contains all your essential amino acids plus antioxidants and omega fatty acids. Many of these plant-based protein powders are awesome not only for providing nutrition but also for reducing inflammation and helping you maintain a healthy immune system. Talk with your healthcare practitioner about which protein powder may be best for you.

Getting to the Gut with Glutamine

Glutamine is an amino acid that's considered essential when the human body is under stress. Glutamine is commonly used in cancer treatments, but it's now being researched and used more to support gut health. From treatment of diarrhea to supporting probiotic health, glutamine is a simple amino acid for you to add to your daily regimen.

An article from the journal *Amino Acids* in 1999 reviewed how essential glutamine is to immune system functioning. Without it, your immune system isn't fully able to supply the body with the immune cells it needs to fight off infections. Therefore, having enough glutamine is essential for successfully fighting off infections.

You can find glutamine in powdered form and add it to water or juice, or you can take it in capsule form. Start with 500 milligrams twice a day, and talk to your healthcare practitioner about when to begin adjusting this dose. Doses at 1,000 milligrams a day have been used to help the body heal during an acute illness or acute injury.

I (coauthor Rich) like to use a plant-based protein powder that contains all the essential amino acids that your body needs, including glutamine (see the preceding section for info on protein powder). I take a protein powder daily.

Powering the Brain with Inositol

Your body makes inositol, so this substance isn't considered an essential vitamin; however, researchers are looking at inositol's role in depression and brain health.

Studies suggest that inositol does your brain a world of good. In studies on depression or bipolar disorder, inositol has been shown to be safe at dosages up to 12 grams per day. Preliminary results of studies on high-dose inositol supplements are promising for treating people suffering from obsessive-compulsive disorder (OCD), bulimia, and panic disorder. Inositol has been well-tolerated with few side effects reported.

Inositol can also boost the immune system. It helps enhance the activity of the natural killer cells and decreases the production of proteins that promote inflammation.

Cantaloupe and oranges are a natural source of inositol, but to receive clinical benefits, it's best to supplement with a pill form. Be sure to consult your physician or dietitian in regard to recommended dosage. It's safe to start at 1 gram per day and work up, based on need.

Because of the connection between gut health and symptoms of depression, coauthor Wendy Jo routinely recommends inositol for her clients, along with probiotics, glutamine, and fish oils.

Correcting Urinary Tract Infections with Cranberry Extract

When the immune system is suppressed, women often find themselves battling urinary tract infections (UTIs). Research shows that mild UTIs can be treated with cranberry extract instead of antibiotics. In addition, cranberry extract has been shown to reduce growth of bad bacteria, such as *E. coli*, *Streptococcus,* and *H. pylori*. You can take cranberry extract in capsule form; take one daily in the morning on an empty stomach.

If yeast infections have plagued you, cranberry extract may offer you relief. One study from the *Journal of Antimicrobial Chemotherapy* in 2009 sought to evaluate the effectiveness of cranberry extract in preventing UTIs. The study participants consisted of 137 women who'd had two or more UTIs that required antibiotic treatment in the past year. The study participants received either trimethoprim (a commonly prescribed antibiotic) or cranberry extract for a period of 6 months.

The authors noted that there was little difference between the efficacy of the antibiotic and the cranberry extract in the prevention of UTIs. They concluded that cranberry extract is an inexpensive alternative that people who've suffered recurrent UTIs should discuss with their healthcare practitioners.

If taking cranberry extract isn't your cup of tea, consider D-mannose as an alternative. D-mannose is the ingredient in cranberry extract that provides relief for recurrent UTIs. This sugar works by coating the bacteria, particularly *E. coli,* to keep them from sticking to the urinary tract. We recommend taking 500 milligrams a day in capsule form.

Chapter 20

Maximizing the Function of Ten Important Organs and Systems

*T*he best way to decrease adrenal stress is to do all you can to keep your body in tiptop shape. A problem with one of your body's organs can adversely affect other organs. When your organs aren't functioning optimally (when they're ill), the adrenal glands are stressed.

This chapter describes ways you can maximize the function of ten important organs and systems. By optimizing the function of your body's organs, you not only reduce your chances of developing adrenal fatigue, but you also increase your body's ability to recover sooner should you develop adrenal fatigue.

You can optimize organ function using various therapies, including supplements and/or mind-body therapies. (As a bonus, when you use natural supplements, you don't just help heal one organ system; you frequently benefit many.)

Before you begin any new supplements or routines, be sure to consult your healthcare provider.

Maximizing Heart Function

The heart is one of the most important organs in the body, so do all you can to maximize your heart function — and in the process, to lengthen your life.

Jump-starting the heart

Your heart is a system based on electrical energy. You want to provide your heart with the energy it needs to function. The heart pumps blood to the adrenals, providing them with the nutrients they need. The last thing you need in the setting of adrenal fatigue is a sluggish heart.

Talk to your healthcare practitioner about adding ubiquinone (coenzyme Q_{10}) and D-ribose to your regimen, especially if you have any history of heart disease or a medical condition (like diabetes or hypertension) that increases the risk of developing heart disease. Flip to Chapter 11 for details on ubiquinone and D-ribose.

Getting the blood flowing to the heart

Part of your strategy for treating adrenal fatigue should be to do everything you can to maximize blood flow to your heart and maintain the pliability of the blood vessels. The following four supplements are invaluable for improving blood flow:

✔ **Vitamin K_2:** This vitamin can help keep calcium from depositing on the heart and blood vessels. It makes no sense to me (coauthor Rich) for millions of people to go in for specialized CT scans just to discover that they have calcium buildup in their vessels. The key is to try to prevent it in the first place. In my practice, I start vitamin K_2 supplementation at 40 micrograms daily.

If you're taking the blood thinner warfarin (Coumadin), you may not be able to take vitamin K_2. Talk with your healthcare practitioner to find out how to proceed.

✔ **Omega-3s:** Not only do omega-3 fish oils lower triglyceride levels, but they can also keep your blood vessels soft and pliable. (High triglyceride levels plus chronic inflammation can increase your risk of developing atherosclerosis, which can decrease blood flow to your heart.) Omega-3s also thin the blood and have a potent anti-inflammatory effect. Begin by taking 1 to 2 grams a day, and talk with your healthcare practitioner before increasing the dose.

✔ **Garlic:** Garlic isn't just for warding off vampires. It also reduces the blood's clotting ability. *Allicin* is a compound in garlic that inhibits vascular calcification, an effect that's important for maximizing blood flow to the heart.

If you buy garlic extract, look for aged garlic extract. You can begin taking 200 milligrams of aged garlic extract once a day; talk with your healthcare provider about adjusting the dose.

✔ **Pomegranate:** Many studies cite the beneficial effects of pomegranate on the heart. For example, an article in the journal *Complementary Therapies in Clinical Practice* in 2011 reviewed the beneficial cardiac effects of pomegranate, including lowering blood pressure and protecting the heart against atherosclerosis.

Pomegranate is such a great antioxidant that I (coauthor Rich) recommend that everyone take it daily. You can obtain this antioxidant in juice or capsule form. Many brands of pomegranate juice are high in sugar, so I tend to recommend the capsules. I take a 500-milligram capsule daily.

Pumping up the heart

Cardiovascular disease is the leading cause of death in industrialized countries, and congestive heart failure (CHF) is the leading reason that people are admitted to the hospital. This is especially true of the elderly population. The two major causes of congestive heart failure are a decrease in the heart's ability to pump blood to the rest of the body (called *systolic* heart failure) and a decrease in the heart's ability to relax (called *diastolic* heart failure).

Congestive heart failure, especially the late stages, can be a source of chronic fatigue in many people. Not only can congestive heart failure contribute to the development of adrenal fatigue, but adrenal fatigue can be harder to recover from if congestive heart failure is present. Some of the medications used to help normalize blood pressure in adrenal fatigue, for example, can't be used in the setting of congestive heart failure. Treating congestive heart failure and maximizing heart function is vital in anyone with adrenal fatigue.

If you've been diagnosed with congestive heart failure, you can take some actions to help your heart pump better. In addition to taking the supplements that you read about in the preceding sections (including ubiquinone, D-ribose, and garlic), you can take hawthorn and arjuna:

✔ **Hawthorn:** This herb helps the heart pump better and has a blood pressure–lowering effect as well. Hawthorn also aids the adrenal glands in hormone production. In fact, hawthorn berries are an ingredient in many supplements that treat adrenal fatigue. I (coauthor Rich) tend to recommend starting at 250 milligrams of hawthorn daily and increasing slowly to 250 milligrams twice a day.

If you're taking the medication digoxin, which is commonly prescribed for congestive heart failure, do not take hawthorn. Hawthorn can increase the levels of digoxin in the blood. When levels of digoxin become too high, they can be toxic. Symptoms of digoxin toxicity include nausea, vomiting, changes in vision, and changes in heart rhythm. Check with your healthcare before taking any other supplements with digoxin, because it can interact with many other supplements and herbs.

✔ **Arjuna:** This herb can help decrease the symptoms of congestive heart failure and can help your heart cope with stress. Arjuna is high in ubiquinone (coenzyme Q_{10}), which may account for some of its heart-healing properties. Consider starting at 400 milligrams a day.

Beating broken-heart syndrome

Broken-heart syndrome (also known as *Takotsubo syndrome*) is an acute enlargement of the heart. It's a cause of congestive heart failure (see the preceding section). Although this syndrome is usually seen in young women, it can occur in men.

In response to acute emotional stress or trauma, the secretion of stress hormones from the adrenal glands increases, affecting the heart's ability to do its job. The adrenal cortex (which we describe in Chapter 2) produces high levels of epinephrine and norepinephrine, which force the heart to work harder. In times of extreme stress, excessive secretion of these hormones can literally cause a broken heart.

How does a heart "break"? The left ventricle, which pumps blood to the rest of the body, can suffer a significant decrease in its pump function. The most common presentation is acute shortness of breath due to *pulmonary edema*, which is fluid buildup in the lungs due to the heart's inability to pump blood.

People do recover from this syndrome, and over time the heart can recover function. This really shows how adrenal and heart function are more closely connected than most people appreciate.

Treating broken-heart syndrome includes stress reduction; meditation; proper nutrition; certain medications that can help the heart function recover (classes of prescription medication such as beta blockers and ACE inhibitors); and supplements, including ubiquinone, D-ribose, pomegranate, and hawthorn.

Taking a Deep Breath: The Lungs

Chronic obstructive pulmonary disease (COPD) is the fourth leading cause of hospital admissions. For many people, especially when they have acute exacerbations of their lung disease (including asthma), the treatment is steroids, given intravenously and then orally. Imagine the long-term effects on the adrenal glands after being on steroids all those years.

Instead of relying on steroids, you can potentially strengthen your lung function. You may be able to decrease or even eliminate the amount of steroids you're taking (and possibly stop using your albuterol inhaler) with the help of the following treatments — and in turn, you can decrease the burden on your adrenal glands. That would be a very good thing.

- **Probiotics:** Probiotics (see Chapter 11) can be especially helpful for kids and adults with asthma. Several studies demonstrate the effects of probiotics in improving asthma symptoms. Probiotics can also be helpful for other lung conditions, including bronchiectasis and cystic fibrosis. I (coauthor Rich) tend to recommend one probiotics capsule daily at a minimum. Some formulations allow you to increase to three times a day. Talk with your healthcare practitioner about the right dose of probiotics for you.

- **Quercetin:** Quercetin (see Chapter 11) can help improve lung function. This is an excellent antioxidant that may help decrease your allergy symptoms as well. Taking 400 milligrams a day can really help improve breathing and decrease shortness of breath.

- **Omega-3 fish oils:** Omega-3s help decrease inflammation. Keep in mind that COPD is an inflammatory process! Begin taking 1,000 to 2,000 milligrams on a daily basis.

- **Resveratrol:** This antioxidant is commonly found in red wine. According to some studies, it can inhibit the lung enzyme *neutrophil elastase* to some degree. This enzyme is responsible for the continued damage in COPD; it eats away at the lung tissue. I tend to recommend starting at a dose of 250 milligrams a day.

- **Magnesium:** Magnesium helps dilate the smooth muscles of the respiratory tract. If you have a lung problem such as COPD or asthma, magnesium deficiency can increase your risk of developing acute attacks. Supplementation (see Chapter 11) should overcome the deficiency.

No Bones about It: The Skeletal System

Just as a well-built house requires a solid foundation, a healthy body requires a solid skeletal system. The skeleton can affect — and be affected by — adrenal fatigue. Excess cortisol secretion from the adrenals over time can cause bone thinning and osteoporosis. An acidic diet increases mineral loss, including calcium and magnesium, and worsens adrenal fatigue.

Maximize skeletal health with supplementation and proper body alignment:

- **Supplementation:** I (coauthor Rich) recommend a good bone mineral supplement that contains vitamins D, C, and K_2; magnesium; calcium; and trace minerals. (Find out more about these vitamins and minerals in Chapter 11.)

- **Body alignment:** A body that's out of alignment can affect adrenal gland functioning. A whole bunch of nerves pass through the bones in your back *(vertebrae)*, which make up the spinal column. If your vertebrae are out of alignment, the condition will likely increase the activity of your sympathetic nervous system (SNS). That amounts to boosting your fight-or-flight reaction, the well-known trigger that releases tons of adrenaline from your adrenal glands. That may increase your blood pressure to levels that are higher than desired and can cause your heart to work really hard. And an unregulated sympathetic nervous system can cause narrowing of the blood vessels *(vasoconstriction)*, which can decrease blood flow to the adrenals.

Your bones can go out of alignment because of bad posture, lifting heavy things without using proper techniques, and sitting in desk chairs all day. Bad footwear, prior back injuries, arthritis, and nerve problems that affect how you walk can add to alignment problems.

A body out of alignment affects more than just your adrenals; you may experience pain anywhere, including in your hips and knees. When you bring your body back into alignment, you'll feel better and help maximize blood and nutrient flow to your adrenal glands.

To check your body's alignment, get a structural examination by a doctor of osteopathic medicine (DO), a chiropractor, or a structural integration specialist.

Seeing Is Believing: The Eyes

The eyes aren't only the keys to the soul; they're also organs affected by adrenal fatigue. Excess cortisol secretion from the adrenal glands over time may contribute to the formation of *cataracts* (clouding of the eye lens). Other medical conditions, including diabetes and certain forms of arthritis, can also affect eye health. Here are three supplements that are beneficial for eye health:

- ✔ **Bilberry extract:** This is an excellent antioxidant for the eyes, especially if you have diabetes.

- ✔ **Vitamin A and the carotenoids:** Vitamin A is the eye vitamin; it's helpful in preserving vision, especially night vision. The carotenoids are also excellent for eyesight; two of them, zeaxanthin and lutein, seem to delay the progression of macular degeneration in some people. (See Chapter 11 for more about vitamin A and carotenoids.)

- ✔ **Omega-3 fish oils:** These have been shown to help promote eye health over time.

Loving the Liver

Think of the liver as the body's processing center. It metabolizes just about everything that enters the body, including medications. To be nontechnical, the liver is your body's toxic waste dump. To be technical, the liver deals 24/7 with *insults,* including deadly poisons, excessive dosages of meds like acetaminophen (in Tylenol), and ethyl alcohol (booze).

Cirrhosis is scarring of the liver. When your liver is damaged, your adrenal glands don't respond to stress the way they need to. Does liver disease affect the ability of the adrenal glands to function optimally? You bet. An article in the *World Journal of Gastroenterology* in 2013 showed that hospitalized patients with cirrhosis didn't have the ability to deal with the acute illness because of their messed-up adrenal glands.

The leading cause of liver disease in the United States is a *fatty liver,* an epidemic condition. Leading risk factors for a fatty liver are obesity and diabetes. If you have either of these two conditions or you use alcohol, consider speaking with your healthcare practitioner about adding the following supplements to improve your liver health:

✔ **Milk thistle:** Many studies show that this herb has protective effects on the liver. Believe it or not, it also has protective effects on the adrenal glands. I (coauthor Rich) tend to start patients on a dose of 100 milligrams twice a day and follow their blood work closely.

✔ **Alpha lipoic acid (thioctic acid):** Many studies point to alpha lipoic acid as having a liver-protective effect. It's one awesome antioxidant (see Chapter 11 for details). I start patients on a very low dose of 200 milligrams a day and increase slowly.

One of the big problems in advanced liver disease is the increased risk of developing low blood sugar levels. The reasons are twofold: First, with cirrhosis, the liver loses its ability over time to help keep up blood sugar levels. I believe that the other reason may be an inadequate response from the adrenal glands, especially if adrenal fatigue or adrenal exhaustion is present. For someone taking alpha lipoic acid, the blood sugar levels need to be followed closely. Alpha lipoic acid can lower blood glucose levels, especially at a higher dosage. That's why I start that supplement at a very low dose of 200 milligrams daily and increase very slowly.

✔ **Probiotics:** Probiotics (see Chapter 11) help a lot of the body's organ systems, including the liver. They help decrease the liver's workload, and that decrease is essential for anyone with liver disease. I recommend taking one minimum dose daily and increasing it to two or three doses daily.

✔ **SAM-e:** Multiple studies demonstrate that SAM-e (S-adenosyl methionine) helps improve liver function. This natural enzyme is present in every cell of the body. I start patients at a very low dose of 200 milligrams daily and increase slowly. By the way, SAM-e also has other benefits, including helping depression and osteoarthritis. *Note:* You should speak with your healthcare provider concerning this supplement if you've ever been diagnosed with Parkinson's or bipolar disorder. Please refer to Chapter 18 for more information on SAM-e.

Supplements alone won't optimize your liver health. Consider lifestyle changes, such as diet and exercise, to give your liver function a boost. Your healthcare professional can advise you.

Knocking Kidney Disease

Kidney disease is the eighth biggest killer in the United States, after heart disease, cancer, respiratory diseases, stroke, accidents, Alzheimer's, and diabetes. Do all you can to keep kidney disease at bay. (In doctor talk, kidney disease is *nephropathy,* which includes *nephrosis* and *nephritis.*)

Because the adrenal glands are so anatomically connected to the kidneys, maintaining kidney health is of the utmost importance for maintaining adrenal health. Here are four things you can do to improve kidney function:

- **Consume a plant-based diet.** Eat your leafy greens, which have a protective effect. (See? Your mother was right when she insisted that you eat your vegetables.) The antioxidants in a plant-based diet can protect the kidneys from the effects of oxidative stress and inflammation.

- **Take your daily probiotic.** There's a significant amount of research on the effects of the immune system on kidney function. Probiotics (see Chapter 11) augment the intestinal microbial population (the gut bugs), and that can help your immune system.

- **Prevent acidosis.** Drinking alkalinized water (see Chapter 11) or taking a bicarbonate supplement may enhance both bone health and kidney health. The kidneys keep the blood alkaline and extract acid, so why overwork them? Vegetables also have an alkalinizing effect.

- **Reduce systemic inflammation.** The kidneys, like other organs, are targets of inflammation. Taking an antioxidant such as turmeric daily should reduce inflammation and therefore (in coauthor Rich's opinion) promote kidney health. Chapter 11 has more about turmeric.

Looking at the Lymphatic System

Everybody talks about blood, but nobody talks about lymph. For shame! The lymphatic system is responsible for processing the waste that builds up in your body. A healthy immune system requires a healthy lymphatic system. A healthy lymphatic system decreases inflammation and adrenal stress. Think of the lymphatic system as (excuse us) the body's septic tank. It needs to be emptied constantly and a healthy flow maintained.

Here are five things you can do to help maintain a healthy lymphatic system:

- **Exercise:** Brisk walking helps improve lymphatic flow. The key is to *move.* (Flip to Chapter 12 for info on exercise.)

- **Massage therapy:** When you get a massage, the practitioner is promoting the movement of the lymphatic system. He or she may say, "I stirred a lot of things up today." That's true, and you'll feel it.

- **Deep breathing:** Many lymph glands are located around the lungs and diaphragm. Breathing deeply with your diaphragm is important in maintaining lymphatic flow. Please see Chapter 6 for the proper way to breathe deeply using your diaphragm.

Restricted diaphragmatic movement can be seen with many lung problems and can directly affect lymphatic flow. If you're seeing an osteopathic physician, ask the doctor about techniques that can help promote lymphatic flow. For example, a technique called the *lymphatic pump* is used to maximize the diaphragm's movement.

If you or a loved one has ever been in the hospital for any medical reason (especially acute lung issues, such as pneumonia or emphysema), you've likely been instructed to use a device called an *incentive spirometer*. This device helps get the diaphragm moving, which improves lymphatic flow. You want to do that so you can get better faster and out of the hospital sooner!

✔ **Hydration:** Maintaining adequate hydration is crucial for maintaining lymphatic flow. Drink six to eight glasses of pure, mineralized water a day. I (coauthor Rich) am a big proponent of alkaline water (see Chapter 11).

✔ **Probiotics:** The small intestine is interconnected with the body's lymphatic system. By helping maintain healthy intestinal flora, probiotics (see Chapter 11) minimize the waste that the lymph glands have to deal with.

Keeping Your Blood in Circulation

In addition to maintaining a healthy blood flow to the heart (which we discuss earlier in this chapter), you want to maintain optimum blood flow to the other organs and your extremities. Here are some natural treatments that can help maximize blood flow:

✔ **Vitamin K_2 and garlic:** Vitamin K_2 and garlic can help maintain healthy blood vessels. Food sources high in vitamin K_2 include leafy greens, including kale and raw parsley.

✔ **Resveratrol:** This potent antioxidant is very helpful for maintaining healthy blood flow. I (coauthor Rich) recommend taking resveratrol in capsule form beginning at 250 milligrams a day.

✔ **Ginkgo biloba:** Extracts from the nuts of this tree can improve blood flow to most tissues and organs. I prefer the capsule form. You can begin at doses as low as 120 milligrams daily.

✔ **Vitamin C:** This vitamin has excellent antioxidant properties for blood vessel health, in addition to being important for adrenal health. Begin at 1,000 milligrams of vitamin C daily. The ester form is absorbed very well.

Thanking the Thyroid

The thyroid gland is often called the *master gland* because it helps keep everything in your body going. It works closely with various organs, including the adrenal glands. Your thyroid controls how quickly your body uses energy, controls how sensitive your body is to other hormones, and makes proteins.

Adrenal fatigue can affect thyroid gland function; the two are intimately related. In the setting of adrenal fatigue, especially in the later stages, your body goes into a sort of self-preservation mode. Adrenal fatigue, inflammation, and acidity wear down the body. As part of this self-preservation, your thyroid gland tries to slow the body down in an attempt to decrease not only adrenal stress but also the effects of adrenal stress on the body. The hope is that by slowing the body down, the body has time to recover.

The thyroid is a significant target for autoimmune disease and inflammation (as are the adrenal glands). Conditions affecting the thyroid tend to have a ripple effect, preventing other organs from functioning optimally. What can you do? Here are some supplements you can use to help maximize thyroid function:

- ✔ **Trace minerals and micronutrients:** Selenium is very important for augmenting thyroid function; see Chapter 11 for more about this and other trace minerals.

- ✔ **Royal jelly:** This is an incredible natural product that I (coauthor Rich) believe has a beneficial effect on thyroid health. It has very potent anti-inflammatory properties that can benefit both the thyroid and the adrenal glands.

When you're beginning to support your thyroid gland, you also need to provide adrenal support, including taking your B and C vitamins (see Chapter 11 for more on these vitamins). These vitamins are crucial for adrenal gland function.

Normalizing the Nervous System

The nervous system is intertwined with the adrenal glands in many ways. The essential fight-or-flight reaction is a stimulation of one aspect of the nervous system (the sympathetic nervous system). The two keys elements in maintaining nervous system health are providing the nutrients that the nervous system needs and calming the system.

- ✔ **B vitamins:** The B vitamins, including B_6 and B_{12} (see Chapter 11), are important not only for adrenal gland health but also for maintaining a healthy nervous system.

- ✔ **Magnesium:** Nerves send messages to each other via a chemical and electrical transmission system. Magnesium and other minerals, such as potassium and calcium (see Chapter 11), are important. Have you ever noticed nerve/muscle twitching (also known as *fasciculations*)? That can point to inadequate magnesium intake.

- ✔ **Aromatherapy with essential oils:** Chamomile oil or lavender oil can help soothe the body and the nerves. Chamomile, in particular, has *anxiolytic* (anti-anxiety) properties that may help reduce stress and insomnia.

Index

About the Authors

Dr. Richard Snyder, DO, is an osteopathic physician who lives in the Lehigh Valley in Pennsylvania. He's a kidney specialist, board certified in both internal medicine and nephrology. He did his Internal Medicine Residency at Abington Memorial Hospital and completed both clinical and research fellowships in nephrology at the Hospital of the University of Pennsylvania. He is a Clinical Professor in Internal Medicine and Nephrology at the Philadelphia College of Osteopathic Medicine. He also has extensive experience in graduate medical education. He is a former Osteopathic Program Director and Associate Program Director of the Internal Medicine Residency Program at Easton Hospital in Easton, PA, where he was responsible for the education of medical residents and medical students. He is currently a Core Faculty Member for their Internal Medicine Residency Program, where in addition to teaching, he serves as Faculty Director of their Clinical Research Program.

In addition to maintaining a clinical practice with St. Luke's Nephrology Associates of St. Luke's University Health Network, he has authored and coauthored several articles in peer-reviewed journals, including the *American Journal of Kidney Disease* and *Kidney International.* He has also presented abstracts at national meetings, including the National Kidney Foundation's Annual Conference. In addition to being a coauthor of *Medical Dosage Calculations For Dummies* and *Physician Assistant Exam For Dummies,* he has authored the books *What You Must Know About Kidney Disease: A Practical Guide to Conventional and Complementary Treatments* and *What You Must Know About Dialysis: The Secrets to Surviving and Thriving on Dialysis.* He has been interviewed regionally and nationally on both radio and television about integrative medicine and kidney disease.

Wendy Jo Peterson, MS, RD, is a registered dietitian with a master's degree in nutritional sciences and is a specialist in sports dietetics. She is the coauthor of *Mediterranean Diet Cookbook For Dummies* and an international speaker, specializing in linking culinary arts and nutrition into a healing plate. She is the owner of a San Diego–based company, Edible Nutrition, and an Austin-based company, Fuelin' Roadie. Find her sharing her exploits, recipes, and quips at www.JustWendyJo.com.

She is a proud military wife and rescuer of black Labs. If she's not in the kitchen, you might be able to find her in the surf or in the mountains, but two things will be certain: She'll be eating well and listening to good music!

Dedication

Rich Snyder: This book I dedicate to my mother, Nancy Snyder, herself a registered nurse and constant source of inspiration and encouragement.

I also dedicate this book to anyone who has ever been told that his or her illness isn't real. We are here to tell you that your symptoms are real, and we are here to help.

I would also like to dedicate this book to Roseanne Silvestri. She is a true example of how one person can make a positive difference in the lives of others. She effects positive change no matter where she is and what she does. That is a true gift.

I finally dedicate this book to a special friend, Father Dan Havron. You took your time to help me once when I really needed it, and you will never be forgotten. You are what I strive to be like on a daily basis.

Wendy Jo Peterson: To my military family, those serving, the ones waiting at home, the widows, and the fallen. We have seen the effects of adrenal fatigue due to a lifetime of war; here's to a future of healing.

And to every physician who takes the time to listen to his or her patients and consider diet as a means of healing them, this book is for you.

Authors' Acknowledgments

Rich Snyder: I would first like to thank Wendy Jo Peterson. She is a wealth of nutritional knowledge and is passionate about helping people. It has been a privilege to work with her on this book. I also need to personally thank Barry Schoenborn. We both were coauthors on my two previous books, and I very much need to thank him for his role as developmental editor for this project. He is an extremely talented writer and editor. I want to thank Tracy Boggier for the opportunity to coauthor this book. I wish to thank Georgette Beatty for her help and support with this book. I want to thank our very talented copy editor, Danielle Voirol. I would like to thank Dr. Jillian Finker, ND, who was the technical editor for the book. I also want to thank Matt Wagner of Fresh Books Literary for the opportunity to write this book.

Wendy Jo Peterson: I cannot thank my coauthor, Dr. Rich Snyder, enough for joining forces with a dietitian on this book. In addition, I'd like to thank my personal physician, Dr. Katie Ballin, for her compassion and beliefs about healing. I'd also like to thank all the physicians I've worked with at San Diego Sports Medicine.

Recipe development and testing is an incredible and joyous task for me, but it's one I couldn't have done without my amazing friends (also known as *recipe testers*): Amy O., Jessica S., Amanda T., Robin S., Erin S., Melanie M., Amanda S., Marisol N., Rachel P., Mahshid S., and Meghann S. Most importantly, thanks to my assistant and intern Danny Sumbillo for his incredible culinary skills and suggestions!

Last but not least, thanks to my husband, my family, and my closest friends, without whose combined support and love my perseverance toward healing people through foods would never be achieved. Thanks, y'all!

Publisher's Acknowledgments

Senior Acquisitions Editor: Tracy Boggier

Senior Project Editor: Georgette Beatty

Senior Copy Editor: Danielle Voirol

Technical Editor: Dr. Jillian Finker, ND

Recipe Tester: Emily Nolan

Nutritional Analyst: Patty Santelli

Art Coordinator: Alicia B. South

Special Help: Barry Schoenborn

Project Coordinator: Patrick Redmond

Illustrators: Kathryn Born, Elizabeth Kurtzman

Cover Image: ©iStockphoto.com/Anna Berkut

Math & Science

Algebra I For Dummies,
2nd Edition
978-0-470-55964-2

Anatomy and Physiology
For Dummies,
2nd Edition
978-0-470-92326-9

Astronomy For Dummies,
3rd Edition
978-1-118-37697-3

Biology For Dummies,
2nd Edition
978-0-470-59875-7

Chemistry For Dummies,
2nd Edition
978-1-1180-0730-3

Pre-Algebra Essentials
For Dummies
978-0-470-61838-7

Microsoft Office

Excel 2013 For Dummies
978-1-118-51012-4

Office 2013 All-in-One
For Dummies
978-1-118-51636-2

PowerPoint 2013
For Dummies
978-1-118-50253-2

Word 2013 For Dummies
978-1-118-49123-2

Music

Blues Harmonica
For Dummies
978-1-118-25269-7

Guitar For Dummies,
3rd Edition
978-1-118-11554-1

iPod & iTunes
For Dummies,
10th Edition
978-1-118-50864-0

Programming

Android Application
Development For
Dummies, 2nd Edition
978-1-118-38710-8

iOS 6 Application
Development For Dummies
978-1-118-50880-0

Java For Dummies,
5th Edition
978-0-470-37173-2

Religion & Inspiration

The Bible For Dummies
978-0-7645-5296-0

Buddhism For Dummies,
2nd Edition
978-1-118-02379-2

Catholicism For Dummies,
2nd Edition
978-1-118-07778-8

Self-Help & Relationships

Bipolar Disorder
For Dummies,
2nd Edition
978-1-118-33882-7

Meditation For Dummies,
3rd Edition
978-1-118-29144-3

Seniors

Computers For Seniors
For Dummies,
3rd Edition
978-1-118-11553-4

iPad For Seniors
For Dummies,
5th Edition
978-1-118-49708-1

Social Security
For Dummies
978-1-118-20573-0

Smartphones & Tablets

Android Phones
For Dummies
978-1-118-16952-0

Kindle Fire HD
For Dummies
978-1-118-42223-6

NOOK HD For Dummies,
Portable Edition
978-1-118-39498-4

Surface For Dummies
978-1-118-49634-3

Test Prep

ACT For Dummies,
5th Edition
978-1-118-01259-8

ASVAB For Dummies,
3rd Edition
978-0-470-63760-9

GRE For Dummies,
7th Edition
978-0-470-88921-3

Officer Candidate Tests,
For Dummies
978-0-470-59876-4

Physician's Assistant Exam
For Dummies
978-1-118-11556-5

Series 7 Exam
For Dummies
978-0-470-09932-2

Windows 8

Windows 8 For Dummies
978-1-118-13461-0

Windows 8 For Dummies,
Book + DVD Bundle
978-1-118-27167-4

Windows 8 All-in-One
For Dummies
978-1-118-11920-4

Available in print and e-book formats.

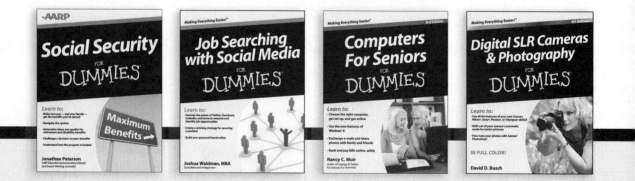

Available wherever books are sold. For more information or to order direct: U.S. customers visit www.Dummies.com or call 1-877-762-2974.
U.K. customers visit www.Wileyeurope.com or call (0) 1243 843291. Canadian customers visit www.Wiley.ca or call 1-800-567-4797.
Connect with us online at www.facebook.com/fordummies or @fordummies

Take Dummies with you everywhere you go!

Whether you're excited about e-books, want more from the web, must have your mobile apps, or swept up in social media, Dummies makes everything easier .

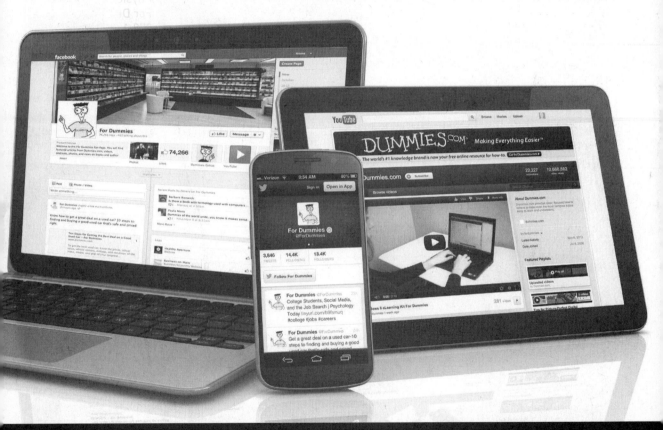

Dummies products make life easier

- DIY
- Consumer Electronics
- Crafts

- Software
- Cookware
- Hobbies

- Videos
- Music
- Games
- and More!

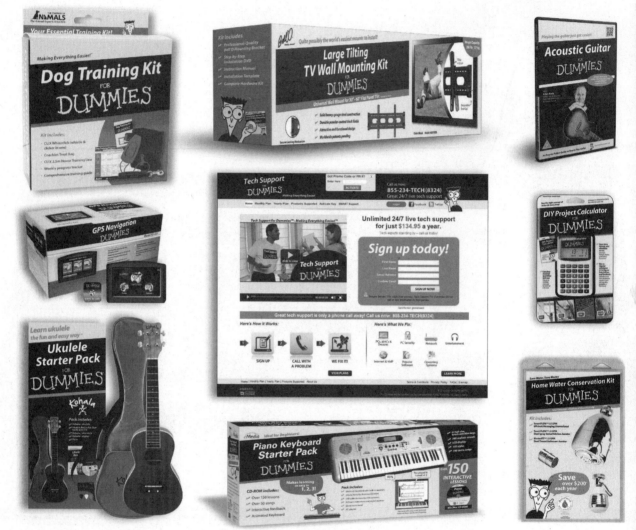

For more information, go to **Dummies.com**® and search the store by category.

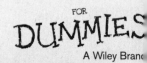